Enriching the Physical Education Service Program in Colleges and Universities

BY

HUBERT J. McCORMICK, Ed.D.

BUREAU OF PUBLICATIONS

Teachers College · Columbia University

NEW YORK, 1942

Preface

THE curriculum content and practices of all fields of education are undergoing critical examination. The purposes of modern education require that traditional practices be re-examined as to educational worth. New courses have been forced into the curriculum by popular demand, by legislative enactment, and by a new, functional concept of education. The curriculum is now overcrowded. Choices must be made regarding the relative worth of content within a given subject matter field, as well as in regard to the values of a given subject as compared to others. Some of the traditional subjects that were formerly required of all students are now offered for a few, some have been dropped entirely from the curriculum, while others have been combined and correlated in the form of introductory or survey courses. Courses lacking in proved educational worth readily apparent in relation to preparation for better living occupy a precarious position in present-day educational programs. Physical education is challenged to demonstrate the values inherent in its practices, not for the few, but for all students.

It is with educational values and the establishment of situations through which these values may be realized by students in the physical education service program that this volume is concerned. Throughout the discussion there are two related themes:

1. That a determination of students' needs is necessary before the content and practices of the physical education service program can be established to prepare students for better living in this area of life.

There are general needs common to all students. These needs constitute the major purposes of this division of education and have long been expressed as objectives, or hoped for outcomes.* Each individual, however, will present his own unique pattern

* See: Chapter I, p. 7.

of needs dependent upon his level of achievement toward a given objective, past experiences in physical education, physical-organic status, occupational choice, and other factors. As needs are determined and situations provided for meeting them, students are thereby better prepared for living.

In the succeeding chapters there will be enumerated a number of technics which can be employed in the physical education service program to determine student needs. There will also be a discussion of a number of student needs which can be served in this field of education. A guidance and advisory plan is indicated whereby each student may draw upon the services of a member of the physical education staff for aid in interpreting needs and choosing a program which best seems to fit these needs.

2. Documentation of the fact that student needs are so numerous and varied that a program of activities alone, no matter how expert the instruction, does not adequately educate students in regard to the backgrounds, purposes, and values of physical education so that they will be sufficiently well informed to make intelligent choices regarding in-school and life pursuits in physical recreational activities.

For this reason it is recommended that the traditional activity program be supplemented with definitely organized instruction concerning the backgrounds, purposes, values, and conduct of physical education. A plan wherein this instruction can be organized and conducted is outlined in the chapters which follow.

Student needs are considered here as the true criteria upon which to establish objectives for the content and practices of the physical education service program. More guidance, both individual and group, is essential in order that students are provided with a background of knowledge and understanding regarding the purposes of physical education and the relative worth of the several activities of the service program. As a result of this adequate guidance the students will be better qualified to make choices in the light of their own unique patterns of needs.

Physical education can be justified in the curriculum of educational institutions only if it prepares students for better living. The acquisition of physical skills in a few athletic sports which are discontinued soon after leaving college is not enough. Students must be prepared to be intelligent spectators as well as skilled participants in many sports and activities, and to understand the place of physical education in their lives. They must be encouraged in the development of knowledge and understandings upon which to base an appreciation of each sport and the broad field of physical education.

Although this book is concerned with the general service program of physical education for all students, the significance and values of related services such as the intramural and intercollegiate athletic programs are not questioned. The point of view here is that they are highly desirable supplements to the broader service program. Any course of study which gives more weight to the intensely spectacular athletic program for the few, to the neglect of the service program for all, may be justly criticized, as indeed many now are. Such an organization of program-making is top-heavy, unstable, and short-sighted of the true purposes of the physical education curriculum. In many colleges adequate service opportunities are not provided for all students. These schools are failing to render the service for which they are established and supported. Many students find it necessary to turn to public, private, and commercial community recreation organizations for the training and experiences which should be afforded by the physical education department as an integral part of their college life.

The physical education service program will be considered, in this investigation, as that part of the physical education course of study commonly known as the "Required Program." It is to be distinguished from other phases of the program such as intramural and intercollegiate athletics, health instruction, and recreation. It is, of course, closely related and contributive to these divisions. The corrective and restricted programs, under whatever terms they may assume, will be considered as a related area of the service program.

Although this book is written primarily with physical education at the college level in mind, many of the proposals for enriching the service program will apply equally well to secondary school physical education programs.

I am deeply indebted to many people who have aided in this study of ways and means whereby the general physical education service program can be organized to better meet the needs of students.

Members of the physical education department of Teachers College, Columbia University, who offered stimulating and helpful advice were Dr. J. F. Williams, Dr. C. L. Brownell, Dr. F. W. Maroney, and Dr. W. L. Hughes. Dr. Hughes also served as my sponsor and was a constant source of inspiration.

Staff members within The Advanced School of Education afforded helpful criticism, both individually and within the graduate seminars and discussions. The approach in terms of student needs was emphasized by Dr. L. Thomas Hopkins. Dr. Carter Alexander was of great assistance in pointing out some of the sources of materials that were used in this study, and was constantly available for helpful and understanding criticism.

Credit is due Arthur L. Acker, Director of Physical Education, Chico State College, who made it administratively possible for much of the material contained herein to be tried and tested within the physical education course of study of that institution.

My wife, Ruth McCormick, has been a continual source of aid and inspiration. Without her assistance the study would never have been attempted. To her, also, credit must be given for preparation of the final manuscript.

While acknowledging this indebtedness I wish to make it clear that any omissions or weaknesses in this final treatment of the problem are the responsibility of myself alone.

HUBERT J. MCCORMICK

Contents

CHAPTER   PAGE

I. INTRODUCTION 1

There is need for an enriched program 1
Aims of the new program 3
Guidance is needed 4
A knowledge of principles is imperative 5
The accepted purposes of physical education indicate
general needs 6

II. TECHNICS FOR DETERMINING STUDENT
NEEDS 10

The health examination is the first essential 11
Records of past experiences 15
The interview 17
Community surveys 20
Observations and rating scales 22
Rating scale for judging performance ability in sports 23
Scales for measuring attitudes and standards of con-
duct 25
Knowledge tests in physical education 28
The use of other types of records and data for deter-
mining student needs 31
Summary 32

III. A FURTHER STATEMENT OF STUDENTS'
NEEDS 33

Proper development and maintenance of the organic
systems of the body 34
Reliable information concerning his own physical-
organic status and the relationship that physical education bears toward the development and maintenance of this status 35
Aid in the development of a philosophy of life 36

vii

CONTENTS

CHAPTER   PAGE

III. A FURTHER STATEMENT OF STUDENTS' NEEDS (*Cont.*)

A knowledge and mastery of the skills, backgrounds, purposes, and values of physical education   37

The ability to handle the body in a well-coordinated manner   38

An understanding of correct body mechanics   39

Qualification as participants and as spectators in many sports   40

Ability to judge success and failure in physical education pursuits in relation to their own individual capacities   43

How to exercise safety precautions in connection with the performance of physical skills   44

An understanding of how games and activities can be modified   46

Proficiency in activities in which they may participate with members of the opposite sex   47

An understanding of the cultural heritage and development of the well-known sports of America   49

In a democracy, students need to learn to lead and to follow as well as to recognize in which of the two capacities they may best serve the group cause   50

Opportunities in which to "forget themselves"   51

Ability to recognize and analyze the claims of fakers, quacks, and physical cultists regarding physical education   52

Development of consumer judgment in relation to the purchase of sports equipment   53

An understanding of the literature of sports and recreation   55

Summary   56

IV. THE SUPPLEMENTARY PROGRAM: ORIENTATION   58

The need for orientation periods   58

The orientation period   60

Content of the orientation period   61

Summary   64

CHAPTER   PAGE

V. THE SUPPLEMENTARY PROGRAM: INTRO-
DUCTIONS AND APPRECIATIONS OF PHYSICAL
EDUCATION 66

The traditional activity program and student needs.. 66
Organization of introductions and appreciations course 70
The teacher 72
How content is determined 73
Summary 79

VI. THE SUPPLEMENTARY PROGRAM: INSTRUC-
TION UNITS 83

An instruction unit in golf 85
An instruction unit in tennis 96

VII. THE ACTIVITY PROGRAM 102

Activities must contribute to needs 102
Criteria for selecting activities 103
Survey courses in activities 108
The syllabus 109
The physical education teacher—an educator 111

VIII. ADMINISTRATIVE PROBLEMS AND PROCE-
DURES 114

The requirement 114
Substitution for the requirement 116
Repeating courses for credit 118
Assigning students to classes 118
The normal or "A" group 119
Restricted and corrective or "B" and "C" groups 119
Program planning 120
Mid-semester changes of program 123
Credit 124
Attendance 124
Marking 125
Library facilities 126

IX. CONCLUSION 128

BIBLIOGRAPHY 132

CHAPTER I

Introduction

There is need for an enriched program

THE college physical education service programs usually reach a large percentage of students. A national survey shows that about 85 percent of the junior colleges, colleges, and universities of America require participation of both men and women in a service program for an average of three hours a week for a period of two years.[1]

In view of the fact that the physical education service program does reach such large numbers of students, it is potentially a great force which can contribute significantly to the life preparation of the young people of America. Education is dynamic. It constantly changes and progresses. A renewed statement of purposes is needed, therefore, for the physical education service program. Traditional practices must be examined and redirected. Regimentation of students into activity sections which produce mere exercise or recreation without regard for the educational values inherent in physical education practices can no longer be condoned. There is need for a clearer statement of purposes in this area of education. As Hughes states:

"The required physical education program is probably the least developed, yet one of the richest in opportunities to students in all higher education. There have been innumerable studies, researches, articles, and convention programs devoted to varsity and intramural athletics, swimming, dance, health instruction, and teacher training; but the service program has remained more or less the uninteresting, unexplored, unimproved, forgotten field."[2]

[1] Rogers, J. F. *Physical Education in Institutions of Higher Education.* Pamphlet No. 82. The United States Office of Education, 1938.
[2] Hughes, W. L. "Enriching the Required Service Program." *The Journal of Health and Physical Education,* p. 205. April, 1939.

1

This statement is significant. The physical education service program, though rich in opportunities, too frequently has been neglected in favor of other divisions of the health and physical education program. A new trend, however, is noticeable. Student needs are being investigated and guidance established in all areas of education. Objectives of education are being stated in a general way. The needs of students are the criteria which indicate the true objectives of physical education for each individual student.

Physical educators are realizing that activity programs for most students have not been organized and conducted with regard for the true purposes of education. It is becoming increasingly apparent that traditional physical education practices have been missing the mark. The needs of students have changed as American society has progressed. The biological unity of man has been irrefutably established.[3] The new organismic psychology, based upon the biological unity of man, indicates the necessity of considering the individual as a whole organism reacting to and affected by its whole environment.[4] An examination of the place of youth in contemporary American society indicates the need for an increased emphasis in regard to leisure and recreative pursuits.[5] The needs of individuals in American society are being examined in the light of pragmatic, functional experimentalism—as this concept has been outlined by Dewey and considered by his colleagues.[6]

[3] Dunbar, H. F. *Emotions and Bodily Changes*. Columbia University Press, New York, 1938.

Cannon, W. B. *The Wisdom of the Body*. W. W. Norton and Co., New York, 1932.

Jennings, H. S. *The Biological Basis of Human Nature*. W. W. Norton and Co., New York, 1930.

[4] Haldane, J. S. *Organism and Environment*. Yale University Press, New Haven, 1930.

Allport, G. W. *Personality—A Psychological Interpretation*. Henry Holt and Co., New York, 1937.

[5] See: American Association of School Administrators. *Youth Education Today*. Sixteenth Yearbook. Washington, D. C., 1938.

[6] Dewey, John. *Experience and Education*. The Macmillan Co., New York, 1938.

Childs, J. L. *Education and the Philosophy of Experimentalism*. The Century Co., New York, 1931.

Rugg, Harold. *Culture and Education in America*. Harcourt, Brace and Co., New York, 1931.

These factors are of significance to physical educators. The actual needs of students in the area of physical education and recreation cannot be met through participation in a program of physical skills alone. Backgrounds, purposes, values, and relationships must be understood. The appreciations, attitudes, and understandings that have long been considered desirable outcomes of physical education are dependent upon a background of knowledge not to be acquired in a program of physical activity alone.

Some physical educators have recognized the need and accepted the challenge. Activity programs have been supplemented with "Orientation" sections. The College Physical Education Association has devoted a section meeting to this problem. Further experimentation has been stimulated, with the result that a few colleges and universities have established a course, which for want of a better term has been called "Orientation in Physical Education."[7]

Aims of the new program

The aims of this new, enriched program in physical education are to be outlined from time to time as this book progresses. These aims serve to indicate some of the needs of students, and to show that frequently the needs which can be met in physical education practices are more than physical. Some general aims are as follows:

1. To "orient" students in regard to the backgrounds, purposes, and values of physical education as well as to certain departmental procedures, facilities, regulations, and services.

2. To lend more meaning and significance to the emerging purposes of students by indicating the relationships of college physical education practices to other courses and practices of

[7] The College Physical Education Association. National Convention in Louisville, Kentucky. W. L. Hughes, Chairman, 1933.

Howard, Glenn. "Enriching Instruction in Physical Education." *Proceedings of the College Physical Education Association,* 1937.

Hermance, Gilbert. "The Nature and Scope of Orientation Courses in Physical Education." *Proceedings of The College Physical Education Association,* 1937.

McCormick, Hubert J. "Orientation in Physical Education." *The Journal of Health and Physical Education,* March, 1940.

the curriculum, particularly to those related areas of health and physical recreation.

3. To make students aware of the aims and objectives of physical education as these apply to each as an individual.

4. To encourage each student to formulate a fact-facing philosophy in regard to health, physical education, and recreation in order that he will be aware of his individual needs to which physical education can contribute.

5. To indicate to students, through individual and group guidance, how physical education can provide situations which will contribute positively to their needs and problems of life which fall within this division of education.

Other aims appear in later chapters. All serve to show that traditional physical education service programs are in need of redirection, and a new statement of purposes is required if the students are to have a well-rounded and balanced program.

Guidance is needed

Physical education needs are many and varied.[8] Some are general for all students; others, more specific for a given individual in relation to his health status and past experiences. Students need help in determining what are their needs. As they become better informed regarding the purposes of physical education, their own individual needs, and the part that certain forms of physical education play in meeting their needs, they will be better qualified to make intelligent choices. Until that time, however, each student should have the advice of a well-qualified physical educator in making out his physical education program. Such guidance is taking an increasingly important part in education. The first principle of guidance involves a purpose on the part of the one seeking aid. Once this purpose is felt, as a definite need, the guide can give personal help. Therefore, the first function of the guide is to be sure that the student himself becomes aware of his needs. The adviser can then assist him in making decisions, in defining purposes, and in learning how best to accomplish these purposes.[9]

[8] See: Chapter III.

[9] Jones, Arthur J. *Principles of Guidance.* McGraw-Hill Book Co., New York, 1934.

Well-qualified teacher-guidance experts are needed in the field of physical education. In addition to mastery of specialized and general subject matter, a working knowledge of guidance technics is required. The teacher-guide must be able to recognize student needs and to help the student make an honest appraisal of these needs. In addition, he must know the relative value of each activity and supplementary instruction situation of the physical education course of study in order to guide students to those situations of most worth to them.[10]

But what are the present needs of college students which can be met through the provision of educative opportunities in the physical education service program? What things can students learn now that will be of practical everyday use to them? In what ways may needs be determined? What administrative measures are necessary for establishing a program that will best meet needs? It is with these and related problems that this book is concerned.

A knowledge of principles is imperative

Before a physical educator can make an objective analysis of the needs of students or the purposes and conduct of physical education, he must have a thorough knowledge and understanding of established principles of physical education. It is not the purpose here to make a detailed statement of principles. This has already been well done in this field of education. Williams' outstanding work has long been recognized as a scholarly and authentic treatment of principles of physical education derived directly from a study of the nature of man—his biological, psychological, and sociological foundations; the place and purposes of physical education in American society; the learning process in physical education; and the derivation of aims and objectives of physical education in the light of data obtained from the study of man, the way he learns, and his place in American society.[11]

Sharman's treatment of principles based upon evidence from

[10] See: Chapter III, p. 36.
[11] Williams, Jesse Feiring. *Principles of Physical Education*. W. B. Saunders Company, Philadelphia, 1938.

biology, psychology, sociology, and education also brings out the backgrounds, purposes, and values of physical education in relation to American life.[12]

A recent publication of The Educational Policies Commission indicates some life needs of students which can be met in the physical education program.[13] Professional literature of the field of physical education is of constant value to those faced with the problem of keeping practices up-to-date.[14] These sources are mentioned for several reasons: rapid progress is being made in physical education, physical educators must be professionally alert if they are to keep abreast of the modern purposes of education as these are outlined in reports of research, experimentation, and the analyses of frontier thinkers. Such sources must continually be consulted if a program which will meet student needs is to be established and maintained.

The accepted purposes of physical education indicate general needs

The purposes of physical education, as they have been stated by experts in the field of physical education, also indicate areas of student need. Such purposes, usually stated in the form of objectives, or hoped-for outcomes, bear out the opinion stated previously that mere physical technics and skills are but one part of the education received through participation in a modern program of physical education. Dr. Williams' statement of objectives has been of great value as a guide to physical educators.[15]

---

[12] Sharman, Jackson. *Modern Principles of Physical Education.* A. S. Barnes and Co., New York, 1937.

[13] The Educational Policies Commission. *The Purposes of Education in American Democracy.* Washington, D. C., 1938.

[14] *The Journal of Health and Physical Education.* Published monthly by The American Association of Health and Physical Education and Recreation. Washington, D. C.

The Research Quarterly. Issued by The American Association of Health and Physical Education and Recreation. Washington, D. C.

Sefton, Alice A. "A Guide to the Literature of Physical Education Including Certain Aspects of Health Education and Recreation." *The Research Quarterly,* Vol. VI, December, 1934.

[15] Williams, Jesse Feiring. *Principles of Physical Education,* Preface, pp. xii–xvii. W. B. Saunders Co., Philadelphia, 1932. Quoted by permission of the publisher.

It holds that the purpose of physical education is the fourfold development of the individual as follows:

1. Development of the organic systems of the individual through physical activities.
2. Development of the neuro-muscular system in general, and particularly in relation to control over certain fundamental skills.
   a. Skills for leisure-time activities.
   b. Skills for safety education.
   c. Skills that are artistic in character, and that afford the performer satisfaction, joy, and pleasure.
3. Development of certain attitudes toward physical activity and particularly toward play. (The development of a philosophy of life which accepts play as a worth-while pursuit.)
4. Development of standards of conduct.
   a. Social standards.
   b. Moral standards.

Similar statements of objectives of physical education are available.[16] These statements are of value in determining a background for a more specific statement of student needs. They represent the opinions of authorities. They are exemplary of experimentalism in that they have been formulated, tried and tested, revised, and re-established as guides to physical education practices.

In connection with the fourfold statement of objectives of physical education which are given above, the following suggested standards will be of value in the interpretation of student needs:

The Objective	Suggested Standards
Organic Vigor	"Normal" for the individual for the ordinary functions of life plus an "emergency reserve."

[16] LaPorte, William R. *The Physical Education Curriculum.* The University of Southern California Press, Los Angeles, Calif., 1940.

Voltmer, E. F. and Esslinger, A. A. *The Organization and Administration of Physical Education,* Chapter III. F. S. Crofts Co., New York, 1938.

The Educational Policies Commission. *The Purposes of Education in American Democracy.* Washington, D. C., 1938.

The Objective	*Suggested Standards (Cont.)*
Neuro-Muscular Skills	Correct form in execution of fundamental skills, such as walking, running, lifting, striking, throwing, catching, etc. This is also a form of safety education.
	Achievement of a level of ability beyond the novice stage in several individual and group activities, some of which will function as adult leisure-time activities.
	Skills that allow the individual to practice self-expression through the medium of bodily activity to the point where joy and satisfaction ensue.
Attitudes	The development by each individual of a fact-facing philosophy of life which accepts "play for the sake of play" as a part of the life plan.
Standards of Conduct	The acquirement of behavior that is acceptable to society and in keeping with that expected of the physically educated man. Such behavior should become habitual with the individual so that it will emerge in any competitive-cooperative situation.
	The conduct should be in relation to the code of ethics unique to the sport in question, whether as participant or spectator.

An examination of these objectives and standards affords a background which serves as a starting point for a further and more detailed investigation into student needs which can be met in the physical education service program. It must be kept in mind in this search for needs that recent evidence shows that learning in physical education is not confined to the acquisition of physical skill. While such skills are being acquired the student also develops attitudes which may be positive or negative in nature, and formulates standards of behavior as one of a social group. In short, the whole individual is learning in a total student-environmental situation. Due attention must be given to this complicated form of learning through experiences. As the statement of student needs progresses it will be found that while physical activity is the principal learning medium in this area of education, there is also a need for learning situations in order to assure that the student is developing understandings and knowledge. In these supplementary situations, it is hoped that the student will attain a background of desirable attitudes and appreciations of physical education.

CHAPTER II

Technics for Determining Student Needs

IF THE physical education service program is to be of real value it must become student-centered and functional. It must first determine the actual needs of students and then provide situations in which these needs can be met. In the previous chapter it was pointed out that an analysis of objectives and standards of physical education affords the initial background material for the determination of general student needs. It is through careful interpretation of data derived from a study of the principles and accepted objectives of physical education that general areas of need for all students are derived. However, the *degree* to which a student has to realize an objective is dependent upon his status at a given time, the scope and degree of his past experiences in physical education pursuits, the play traditions and customs of the particular region or community in which he is preparing to live, the type of life work he plans to pursue, and other factors which will appear as the analysis of student needs progresses.

It is important to remember that although all students have needs in general, the status of each as an individual must be determined before any specific objective to be realized in the service program is set up. Any other procedure is of doubtful educational value and leads to regimentation and the traditional assignment to classes without regard for the individual. On the other hand, students must learn to accept, as their own, certain objectives which seem to fit their particular needs. This is necessary in order that they may have a starting point of an individual purpose or plan. Without this plan or purpose, they will achieve little ability for self-direction while in school or as adults.[1]

Students, therefore, must become aware of their own needs, learn to distinguish between fleeting interests and actual enduring needs, be aided to set up a plan of participation in situations which will best contribute to these needs, and be allowed increasing self-responsibility to set up their own programs in the field of physical education.

The following technics will aid in determining the status of each student and the needs which can be met by the physical education service program.

The health examination is the first essential

A thorough health examination will reveal the individual's physical and organic status. It should be the first device used in the determination of student needs, and no assignment to activity should be made without full health examination data. The examination should include heart, lungs, vision, hearing, teeth, nose, throat, nutrition, skin, feet, spinal deviation, general posture, height, weight, and a historical record of diseases and of serious injuries (especially cranial injuries). As a result of the examination some students will be found without defects of such nature as to limit their participation in any phase of the physical education program. These students should be classified in the "A" group.[2] Other students will be found with certain temporary or permanent conditions which limit the amount of activity and the strenuousness of participation. These students would be classified as "Restrictive or Modified Cases" and would include convalescent or rest cases who are permitted to participate in very minor activities only. Students in this group should be classified as the "B" group.

[1] See: Caswell, H. L. and Campbell, D. S. *Curriculum Development*, Chapter VI. American Book Co., New York, 1935. An excellent discussion of the aims of education and how they are derived.

[2] The A, B, C classification recommended here is in keeping with the recommendation of The Committee on Curriculum Research of the College Physical Education Association. See: *The Physical Education Curriculum*, pp. 45–46. The University of Southern California Press, Los Angeles, 1940.

Some students will be found with conditions that seem possible of improvement to some degree. These students are to be considered as "Corrective Cases." Students in this group would fall in the "C" classification. In some situations, students in the "B" and "C" groups can be sectioned together for modified activities. It is agreed that, whenever possible, students in these classifications should take part in many of the same activities as students in the regular classification. Of course the degree of activity must be modified so that there is no chance of aggravating the condition of these students. Restricted students need an understanding and an appreciation of many games, as well as the regular students, and should not be denied opportunities of safe participation in modified game forms.

The obligation to students does not cease upon assignment to any one of the above groups and the outlining of a program of activities. Other needs must be served. Students need to know what is the meaning of "normal" according to the results of the examination, how this level is achieved, how it can be retained, and how it is approached after one has gotten "out of condition." These needs will fall under the following heads:

1. To understand the relationship of organic vigor to health.

2. To understand that organic vitality is developed and maintained only through vigorous physical activity.

3. To be aware of safety, sanitary, and hygienic practices connected with physical education and their importance for the maintenance of a sound physical and organic condition.

Students in the restricted and corrective classifications also have needs in relation to their conditions. In addition to the foregoing, they need:

1. To have a thorough and accurate knowledge of their condition and the causes thereof.

2. To know if the condition is temporary or permanent and, if temporary, how to approach "normal" as soon as possible.

3. To know what types and degrees of participation are physically wholesome for them.

4. To be able to recognize signs of fatigue, know when they are running a chance of aggravating their condition, and regulate their activities accordingly.

5. To be aided in the development of a philosophy which faces the facts, yet points out to them that they can live a relatively full life in spite of their condition.

Students should be assigned to those activities of the physical education program which the findings of the health examination indicate are best suited to them. The health examination will reveal many general as well as individual needs of particular students. The physical educator will assign the students in the regular classification to any activity of the program. But students in the restrictive or corrective classifications must be assigned to activities upon the recommendation of the school health officer. The physical educator has no legal right to diagnose defects or prescribe treatment therefor. He will be expected, however, to be intelligent enough to supervise a program which has been laid out in cooperation with the school health officer.

The health examination, then, will indicate some needs of students. But there are many other areas of student need. Further technics will help to reveal them.

It is recommended that at the time of the health examination a physical education classification card (Table I) be filled out and sent to the director of physical education. In order to facilitate the filing of these cards it is suggested that several colors be used: white for the normal students, blue for the restricted students, and red for the corrective students. All students who have been excluded from school because of illness or injury should be required to obtain a readmittance slip from the health officer's office, and if necessary, to receive a change of classification.

The health examination is to be required of all new students, and may be used as an administrative device at this time. As each new student is examined he should be assigned to a staff member of the physical education department as his adviser. The apportionment of students to an adviser should be equalized. Students in the "B" and "C" classifications should go to

TABLE I

PHYSICAL EDUCATION CLASSIFICATION RECORD

"A" Classification

.... has been examined and comes within the "A" classification.

Examined by .... Date ....

Remarks:

Adviser Assigned: ....

"B" Classification

.... has been examined and comes within the "B" classification.

Examined by .... Date ....

Remarks:

This student has an "adolescent heart." Modified activity under controlled conditions will benefit him. He must not take part in highly competitive games, such as basketball, touch football, running events in track, or similar activities. He has been informed in regard to his condition, its cause, and how to recognize signs of fatigue in relation to the condition.

Re-examination recommended for: *Immediately after Christmas Holidays*

Adviser Assigned: ....

"C" Classification

.... has been examined and comes within the "C" classification.

Examined by .... Date ....

Remarks:

The program for this student may be made out only after a personal interview with the medical officer.

Adviser Assigned: ....

the director of that phase of the program—in those institutions large enough to justify a staff member in charge of restricted and corrective cases.[3] These "B" and "C" students are also assigned to the school physician. He and the delegated staff member act as advisers, and the program is laid out for students in relation to their special needs.

Records of past experiences

In order to further determine needs of students it is necessary to know something of their past experiences in physical education, recreation, and athletics. The service program is concerned with skills, knowledge, attitudes, and appreciations that students may have acquired in many activities. Physical educators know that team games are high in potentiality for developing social skills, such as the ability of getting along with others, cooperation, sportsmanship, leadership. But they also know that team games usually are not very significant as carry-over activities into adult life. (See Table II.) It is also known that many individual sports, while not presenting situations high in the possibility of developing social qualities, are on the other hand high in carry-over value. It seems desirable, then, that the needs of college students for a reasonable degree of skill, for adequate knowledge, and for suitable appreciation of some team games and some individual activities be recognized. It has been suggested that each college man should become skilled in at least two individual sports and two team sports.[4]

If a student, however, has already participated in a number of sports in high school, or in community recreation pursuits, it is doubtful if he should be allowed to duplicate a performance of these activities for college credit. The service program is not merely a recreation program. It would be more in keeping with the needs of the student if he were encouraged to take part in other sports of the program with which students and adults should be familiar. Instruction in game skills and the develop-

[3] See: Chapter VIII.
[4] Hughes, W. L. *The Administration of Health and Physical Education for Men in Colleges and Universities*, p. 70. Bureau of Publications, Teachers College, Columbia University, New York, 1932.

ment of a knowledge and appreciation of many activities should be a part of the service program. Students will then actually be preparing for a more intelligent life in regard to recreation, as participants and onlookers.

As skills and appreciations are developed students should be

TABLE II

CARRY-OVER EXPECTANCY IN PHYSICAL EDUCATION ACTIVITIES
FOR THE AVERAGE MAN

Activity	Graduation	25	30	35	40	50	Life
Basketball		x					
Touch football	x						
Speedball	x						
Soccer	x						
Softball				x			
Track and field	x						
Handball				x			
Volleyball					x		
Tennis						x	
Badminton					x		
Boxing		x					
Wrestling	x						
Tumbling	x						
Swimming							x
Golf							x
Bowling							x
Winter sports							x
Outdoor activities:							
Hunting							x
Fishing							x
Hiking							x
Camping							x
Woodcrafts							x
Boating							x
Riding							x
Cycling							x
Archery							x
Fencing							x
Horseshoes							x
Social dancing							x
Squash				x			
Table tennis							x

Note: This table is a rough approximation. Individual interests, physical condition, etc., will modify it.

encouraged to continue to participate in activities that are afforded in the athletic and intramural programs. However, they should no longer receive credit for this recreational program.

The data concerning the past experiences of students in physical education and recreational pursuits should be recorded on a permanent record form. (Table III.) As the physical education adviser helps the student make up his program this record form should be consulted and kept up-to-date. It will indicate the degree of balance between team and individual activities, will show at once desirable activities in which the student should be encouraged to participate, and will serve as a place for recording other significant data which may be used in guiding students. For example, it should include data from the personnel record of the dean's or guidance department's office, aptitude scores and scores received in attitude ratings in physical education, the health examination data, and the life work the student proposes to take up. All of this comprises significant data for the staff member who is to aid the student to choose physical education experiences in relation to needs. It would also be worth while to record on this form any information that may be acquired by means of surveys after the student has completed his college work.

It is best to have each student aid the instructor in filling out the record card. This can be done by means of interviews.[5] The recording will throw light on the past experiences in physical education, will indicate the present needs of the student in physical education, and will chart a course for the future. The record cards over a period of time will become very valuable for purposes of research.

The interview

The interview is another technic through which the needs of students may be determined. Interviews are of two types, generally speaking: the planned interview, in which a definite time is appointed; and the casual interview, which may take place

[5] See: Chapter VIII.

TABLE III

PHYSICAL EDUCATION CUMULATIVE RECORD CARD

Name: .... High school graduated from: ....

Date of graduation: .... Age: .... Height: .... Weight: ....

Class: .... Proposed life occupation: ....

Years expect to attend college: .... Health classification: A .... B .... C ....

Physical education adviser: ....

Remarks concerning health status in relation to physical education program:

Activities in High School (Student should name activities he liked best in high school physical education)	Individual	Team	As Member of Varsity Team (or Intramural)
	1.	1.	1.
	2.	2.	2.
	3.	3.	3.
	4.	4.	4.
	5.	5.	5.
	6.	6.	6.
	7.	7.	7.
	8.	8.	8.

In what activities would student like to have instruction in the college physical education program?	1.	1.	1.
	2.	2.	2.
	3.	3.	3.
	4.	4.	4.
	5.	5.	5.

What activities does the student take part in during after-school hours, vacation periods, etc.?	1.	1.	On a Club Team
	2.	2.	1.
	3.	3.	2.
	4.	4.	3.
	5.	5.	4.

Adviser's recommendation for activities in the service program. (In rank order)	1st. Sem.	2nd. Sem.	3rd. Sem.	4th. Sem.
	1.	1.	1.	1.
	2.	2.	2.	2.
	3.	3.	3.	3.

Comments regarding the student's particular pattern of needs and guidance program suggested.

Other Data: Results of aptitude, intelligence, and other tests given in other departments of the institution.

Note: On reverse side of this card student's semester marks may be recorded, together with remarks and statements of need and achievement. (Table IX, p. 126.)

before or after class, during the shower period, or in similar informal circumstances where the student and a staff member may be together. Strang says:

"Although success in interviewing cannot be acquired by reading a book on the subject, any personnel worker can improve his technique by a combination of study, practice, and critical evaluation of his procedure."[6]

Many physical educators are expert in interviewing. All can develop and improve in the use of the technic. It must be remembered that the planned interview should not be an ordeal for the student. It should, rather, afford an opportunity for a staff member to gain an insight into the past experiences of the student in the area of recreation and physical education. The student, upon the close of an interview, should emerge with a clearer understanding of his problems in the field of physical education and recreation, with a new interpretation of the place of physical education in preparing him for life, with a feeling of satisfaction that he is being considered as an individual student, and perhaps with a plan in mind resulting from this new evaluation.

It has been recommended that staff members be assigned certain students whom they are to interview and advise. All new students should be interviewed and a record of their past experiences obtained before they are permanently assigned to any physical education section. Students who seem to have difficulty in adjusting themselves in the physical education program should be re-interviewed in order to discover what their individual difficulties are. An interview of from ten to fifteen minutes may yield valuable information in regard to individual needs. By spreading this responsibility to each member of the staff it becomes administratively possible to make more use of this valuable technic in the service program of physical education. If appointments cannot be arranged for individual conferences or interviews, it is possible to assemble small groups of students to point out the objectives of the service program,

6 Strang, Ruth. *Counseling Technics in College and Secondary School*, p. 52. Harper and Brothers, New York, 1937.

to bring out a few of the thought-provoking problems that are common to most students, and then to have each student make out his own card with close supervision of the staff member in charge. As students become better informed about their needs, learn to understand and to appreciate the purposes and values of physical education, and therefore to become more self-directive, the need for interviews will diminish.

Community surveys

Another means of determining the needs of students is the community survey. It must be kept in mind that the term community has come to have a much broader meaning in recent years. The ease of transportation, the opening up of summer and winter wonderlands by the United States Forest and Park Services, and the rise of private and community camps—all must be considered when the term is used in connection with physical education and recreation pursuits.

Two types of surveys are of value to physical educators: the first, a survey of play areas, facilities, and equipment in the community which provide out-of-school play opportunities for students and adults; the second, a survey of the play interests of students and adults in the community which the school serves. These two types of surveys can be conducted by one of the following procedures:

1. List all available play areas, facilities, athletic clubs, sports leagues, winter sports areas, aquatic areas, community recreation facilities and other facilities available to students after school, during holiday and vacation periods, and upon graduation. Determine the popular activities in each instance. Then include instruction in these activities in the service program as representative of the activities students will have an opportunity to participate in as part of their community life.

2. Obtain surveys of the recreational interests of large numbers of people wherever such surveys have been conducted and compare them with the best available information concerning such interests in the local community. This procedure is of some value, but careful consideration must be given to differ-

ences in locality, typography, climate, play traditions, interests of participants, and similar factors.

3. Conduct periodical surveys of the recreational interests of ex-students and graduates of the college. Haynes[7] in a study of the interests of 400 graduate students of Stephens College collected data that resulted in some changes in the physical education course of study. Golf was added and an additional emphasis was placed upon tennis and swimming, as a reasonable proficiency in these sports was listed as a need of these graduates. Scott[8] used this technic in questioning 990 business men regarding their recreational interests, and reports that swimming, fishing, golf, hiking, gardening, hunting, calisthenics, tennis, handball, and volleyball—in that order—were best liked and most often participated in as leisure-time pursuits.

4. Determine the recreational interests of the students now in attendance at college. These data should be included on the record card, discussed under the heading of past experiences. Davis[9] upon the completion of such a study concluded: "That the completed study represents one way of making one step in the selection of content of the required physical education program and the method of teaching it."

The survey is of considerable worth as one means of determining students' needs. It must be pointed out, however, that it merely reveals the status quo, or current interests. It is subject to the same criticism that has always been directed at student interests as determiners of course content—namely, that interests are dependent upon past experiences. Physical education, if it is to be progressive, must always be alert to trends which may not be revealed through student interests alone. Then, too, interests do not always reflect actual needs.

Such surveys, though, are of value when used with other needs-determining procedures. The survey technic can be of much value in pointing out some of the needs of college students. A

7 Haynes, Wilma. "After College, What?" *The Research Quarterly*, March, 1931.

8 Scott, Harry A. "Physical Education and Exercises for Business Men." *The Nation's Health*, June, 1927.

9 Davis, E. C. "A Study of the Interests of Pennsylvania State College Freshmen in Certain Formal and Natural Physical Activities." *The Research Quarterly*, December, 1933, pp. 49–50.

survey of the graduates of a given college, for example, once every four years, will indicate the interests of graduates for each generation of college students and be of value in suggesting program content and method. Colleges and universities with graduate teacher-training departments in physical education might well have students conduct such surveys once every four years as subjects for Master's theses. Comparisons would undoubtedly indicate significant trends of interest to those in charge of the service program and would be of considerable value to the profession as a whole. It is recommended that, wherever possible, community surveys be conducted, the results be tabulated and interpreted, and the service program be redirected if the survey findings indicate that this is desirable.

Observations and rating scales

Another technic of value in determining student needs is the use of observation and rating scales. Strang[10] points out that the reliability of observation ranges from practically zero in the case of casual observations of the untrained teacher to almost perfect positive correlation in the case of observation of a specific kind of behavior by a well-trained observer. The technic of observation is valuable in that it takes into account the "whole situation"; that is, it affords a judgment of the student's behavior in actual game participation and does not measure merely performance in an isolated skill. It contrasts the possession of mere knowledge of proper standards of conduct with the practice, or similar factors completely isolated from the whole situations in which they commonly occur.

Experienced physical educators, and particularly those who have had coaching experience, are usually trained in the technic of observation. Experience in the use of this technic will increase the ability to observe and make sound interpretations in regard to students' needs. Observation results, when combined with other data to be found on the record card of each student, will reveal valuable information concerning a student's behavior which, when translated into terms of his needs, will indicate

[10] Strang, Ruth. *Op. cit.*, p. 94.

specific physical education situations to be conducted to meet these needs. The good observer should possess the following qualities:

1. Be free from bias.

2. Have a background of knowledge that will prevent his interpretation from being naive and superficial.

3. Be able to record results simply, in usable form, and with economy of time.

4. Be able to supplement observational ratings with other technics and records.

5. Keep an average or superior standard of behavior in mind as a basis upon which to make ratings.

Most any area of behavior can be judged by the use of the observation technic along with rating scales. Its use is recommended to physical educators as a device which will aid them in making more objective ratings of judgments, which must be made anyway. If a scale is used, the observation is bound to become more objective than the daily judgments that are made of a student's behavior in various situations of the program. Rating scales are of value for judging performance in physical education activities, for making a rating of attitudes as these are reflected in behavior in game situations, and for determining to what extent knowledge of desirable standards of conduct is actually put into effect in activity situations.

RATING SCALE FOR JUDGING PERFORMANCE ABILITY IN SPORTS

Physical educators have been concerned for a long time about the measurement of individual and team skills. Many tests have been devised which measure individual skills.[11] One objection

11 For examples of skill tests see:
Bovard, J. F. and Cozens, F. W. *Tests and Measurements in Physical Education,* especially Chapters VII and XI. W. B. Saunders Company, Philadelphia, 1938.
Cozens, F. W. *Achievement Scales in Physical Education Activities for College Men.* Lea and Febiger, Philadelphia, 1936.
Glassow, R. B. and Broer, M. A. *Measuring Achievement in Physical Education.* W. B. Saunders Company, Philadelphia, 1938.
Also: Current issues of *The Research Quarterly.*

TABLE IV

BASKETBALL RATING CHART*

Name: .... Age: .... Height: .... Weight: .... Date:				
Game Skills	Excellent	Good	Fair	Poor	Remarks
Passing				
Push				
Overhead				
Bounce				
Right hand				
Left hand				
Shooting				
Close set-ups				
Long shots				
Free throws				
General Coordination				
Controlled Speed				
Dribbling				
Pivoting				
Feinting				
Aggressiveness				
Ball Handling				
Ability to Get Rebounds				
Team Play (Cooperativeness)				
Sportsmanship				
Physical Condition				
Others				
Remarks and Recommendations				

* *Directions for marking:*

EXCELLENT: Full mastery of the fundamentals. A team player with possibility of qualifying as varsity caliber. Not in need of instruction on the service program level. Largely self-directive in basketball. Might serve as student leader or assistant coach.

GOOD: Good mastery of fundamentals. Has room for improvement through instruction and participation. A better than average player but not as finished as the "Excellent" player. Probably of intramural caliber.

FAIR: Capable of playing well enough to derive enjoyment and satisfaction therefrom. Has enough mastery of fundamentals and team play to benefit quickly and definitely from further instruction and participation.

POOR: Poor neuro-muscular coordination. Not sufficient mastery of fundamentals to derive satisfaction from play. Should receive enough instruction and opportunity to play to verify the rating as well as to gain a first-hand appreciation of the game. If he does not show improvement he should be encouraged to take up other activities in which he is more likely to succeed.

to them is that the ability to perform a given skill, isolated from the many other elements that go to make up an all-round successful performance, is not reliable for predicting possible success in an actual whole activity situation. Even if such tests are used it is wise to supplement them with the technic of observation and of rating scales in order to get a true picture of student performance. By means of this technic it is possible to make a fairly objective judgment of individual skills *while the individual is making use of them in a whole situation.*

A rating chart which can be used for recording performance of skills in basketball is shown in Table IV. Similar scales can be constructed for any physical education activity, individual or team. Judicious use of such rating scales will provide the physical educator with much significant data. They will point out student needs in regard to the performance of individual skills in game situations, and will indicate the display of sportsmanship, cooperation, team play, and other qualities.

SCALES FOR MEASURING ATTITUDES AND STANDARDS OF CONDUCT

Some of the most significant learnings to be achieved in physical education are the attitudes and standards of conduct that students accept and put into practice. Indeed, the degree to which skills and physical-organic needs will continue to be affected by life participation in activities is directly dependent upon the attitudes the student develops regarding continued participation in them—quite as much as upon the skill achieved in them. Two of the four major objectives of physical education proposed by Williams[12] and accepted generally by the profession deal with attitudes and standards of conduct. The most objective way of judging attitudes and standards of conduct, as these are accepted and put into practice by students, is by observation in actual activity situations; for it is what the student *practices* and *omits* that charts his needs in regard to further development.

A carefully constructed rating scale will aid in looking for specific traits and afford a means of making comparative judgments. For example, a scale designed to check specific traits is

[12] Williams, Jesse Feiring. *Op. cit.*, 1938, Chapter XIII.

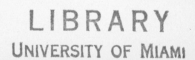

TABLE V

A BEHAVIOR FREQUENCY RATING SCALE FOR THE MEASUREMENT OF CHARACTER AND PERSONALITY IN PHYSICAL EDUCATION CLASSROOM SITUATIONS*

Name of person rated: .... Grade: .... Age: ....
Name of rater: .... Date: ....

Directions: Encircle the number value which best rates the student on that quality. Insert the letter "N" for No Opportunity to Observe.

	No opportunity to observe	Never	Seldom	Fairly Often	Frequently	Extremely Often	Score
Leadership							
1. He is popular with classmates		1	2	3	4	5	
2. He seeks responsibility in the classroom		1	2	3	4	5	
3. He shows intellectual leadership in the classroom		1	2	3	4	5	
Positive Active Qualities							
4. He quits on tasks requiring perseverance		5	4	3	2	1	
5. He acts aggressive in his relations with others		1	2	3	4	5	
6. He shows initiative in assuming responsibility in unfamiliar situations		1	2	3	4	5	
7. He is alert to new opportunities		1	2	3	4	5	
Positive Mental Qualities							
8. He shows keenness of mind		1	2	3	4	5	
9. He volunteers ideas		1	2	3	4	5	
Self-Control							
10. He grumbles over decisions of classmates		5	4	3	2	1	
11. He takes a justified decision by teacher or classmates without anger		1	2	3	4	5	

* Blanchard, B. E. "A Behavior Frequency Rating Scale for the Measurement of Character and Personality in Physical Education Classroom Situations." *The Research Quarterly*, October, 1930. Reproduced with the permission of the publisher and the author.

TABLE V (*Continued*)

	No opportunity to observe	Never	Seldom	Fairly Often	Frequently	Extremely Often	Score
Cooperation							
12. He is loyal to his group		1	2	3	4	5	
13. He discharges group responsibilities well		1	2	3	4	5	
14. Cooperative in attitude toward teacher		1	2	3	4	5	
Social Action Standards							
15. He makes loudmouthed criticisms and comments		5	4	3	2	1	
16. He respects the rights of others		1	2	3	4	5	
Ethical Social Qualities							
17. He cheats		5	4	3	2	1	
18. He is truthful		1	2	3	4	5	
Qualities of Efficiency							
19. Seems satisfied to "get by" with tasks assigned		5	4	3	2	1	
20. Is dependable and trustworthy		1	2	3	4	5	
21. He has good study habits		1	2	3	4	5	
Sociability							
22. He is liked by others		1	2	3	4	5	
23. He makes a friendly approach to others in the group		1	2	3	4	5	
24. He is friendly		1	2	3	4	5	

General Remarks:

Blanchard's revision of a rating scale originally devised by McCloy.[13] (See Table V.)

The use of such personnel rating scales will make the service program a better place to serve the needs of students in the development of desirable attitudes and standards of conduct. One rating of a student's behavior is of some value, but several ratings are desirable. Making several ratings in different activity situations will determine if the sample taken of student behavior truly shows that standards of conduct have been *generally* accepted for all situations, or if one particular type of activity results in a different standard of behavior from that in another. In time, results of such ratings will serve as excellent research material. There should be further research in this area of physical education. Such scales as illustrated here, however, have been and will continue to be of great value in the determination of student needs.

Knowledge tests in physical education

The term "appreciations" is used quite extensively in the literature of physical education. Appreciations of many kinds are considered in this study to be needs of students.[14]

Knowledge tests are one means of determining whether or not students are developing the background necessary for desired appreciations. While it is true that knowledge in itself is of little value to a student until it is made use of in practice, it is equally true that there can be no appreciation of a performance without a background of knowledge of that performance. For instance, a student cannot have an appreciation of the place that physical education should have in his life until he has a knowledge of the benefits that can be derived through lifetime physical education practices. Knowledge, then, is essential for appreciation. It lends significance to the doing. It reveals the "why" phase of an activity situation as well as the "how." Football coaches consider the "why" phase absolutely essential. Consequently they

[13] McCloy, C. H. "Character Building through Physical Education." *The Research Quarterly*, October, 1930, pp. 41–61.
[14] See: Chapter III.

conduct "skull sessions," give examinations on the daily material, the skills and fundamentals, when a particular skill should be brought into play, the defense for a particular offense and vice versa, strategy of the game, and many related factors. The service program likewise must include significant learnings that can be brought about by means of lectures, discussions, illustrations, demonstrations, the use of motion pictures and other supplements to the activity program.

While knowledge tests will reveal needs, they will at the same time contribute to the student's understanding. The results, too, will be an important item in the objective marking procedure.

There is much material in connection with physical education and recreation with which students must become familiar if they are to be qualified as "physically educated." Several general fields of student needs for knowledge seem to be:[15]

1. A knowledge of the place of physical education in one's life.

2. A knowledge of the need for vigorous physical activity for the development of that organic vitality which is the basis of health.

3. A knowledge of the origin, history, development, and worth of the many activities of physical education.

4. A working knowledge of the rules and regulations of many of the games and contests which go to make up a repertoire of adult recreation—both as participant and as spectator.

5. A knowledge of how to "condition one's self" for participation in strenuous activity, how to maintain this condition, how to avoid accidents and injuries in connection with each activity, and how to care for one's self in the event of injury and accident.

Other areas in which students should have a working knowledge are discussed in chapters to follow. It is proposed here that the degree of knowledge a student has is a direct conditioner of the degree of appreciation he can develop in regard to desirable learnings in physical education.

Knowledge tests can be constructed in connection with game skills that are covered in activity programs, upon material dis-

15 See: Chapters III and V.

cussed in lecture and laboratory periods, upon material in the daily sport pages, or upon incidents of the last home football, basketball, baseball, or other contest. The following is suggested as a sample:

Directions: Some of the following statements are true and some are false. If the statement is true, place the letter "T" before it; if the statement is false, or partly false, place the letter "F" before it. Answer all statements. One point will be deducted for each statement answered incorrectly.

Statements regarding Game Skills

1. The overlapping grip in golf undoubtedly affords better control of the club than the interlocking grip.
2. Keeping the eye on the ball during the swing is a rule of golf which should never be violated.
3. Coordinated footwork is an essential part of the "set up shot" in basketball.
4. A defensive player in basketball should keep the feet close together so that he will be taller, and consequently more difficult to shoot over.
5. The side stroke, properly executed, finds the swimmer looking back over the upper shoulder.
6. In the American Crawl, the swimmer should get a complete breath with every complete stroke.
7. The short, from behind the ear, throw in football is faster and more accurate than the long "wind up" type of throw.
8. The offensive line in football should always charge hard regardless of whether the play is a pass, punt, or run.
9. In hitting a baseball it is best to make the swing of the bat parallel to the ground.
10. In catching a baseball the arms and hands should be held rigid in readiness for the shock of the catch.

Statements regarding Knowledge (or Materials) upon Which to Develop an Appreciation of Games

1. A celebration commemorating the 100th anniversary of baseball was held at Cooperstown, New York, in 1939.
2. Basketball was played originally in Germany and came to America from that source.
3. In golf, par is determined by the distance and difficulty of a given hole, and par for a hole is never more than 5.
4. Our varsity basketball team uses a zone defense exclusively.
5. The World's record in the 100-yard dash is held by Glenn Cunningham at 9.3 seconds.
6. The sport of Badminton is named after an English estate by that name.
7. The 6-2-2-1 defense in football appears to be the one most commonly used at the present time.
8. One may approach the green in golf as soon as the group ahead has started putting.
9. The spectator's codes of conduct for baseball and tennis have traditionally assumed different roles.

10. From an educational point of view, the learning of proper golf etiquette is quite as important as the acquisition of skill in the game.

Statements regarding Physical Education as a Life Pursuit
 1. Organic vitality can only be achieved through vigorous big-muscle activity.
 2. The breathing exercises broadcast over the morning radio are undoubtedly of great benefit to all of those who participate in them.
 3. The more skill one has in an activity, the better one likes to participate in it.
 4. The "warm-up period" before an athletic contest results in the attainment of "second wind" before the contest starts.
 5. Present-day emphasis upon leisure time makes a knowledge of desirable leisure-time pursuits an obligation of every educated man.
 6. There are no reliable reasons why women should not take part in the same physical education activities that men do, and if the women are strong and vigorous they should be encouraged to participate with the men.
 7. The process of "handicapping" makes it possible to equalize two players of different ability in golf so that a fair match can be played between them.
 8. The teaching of physical education in schools is educationally justifiable only if students have opportunities to learn things which they can continue to make use of when out-of-school.
 9. One should have sufficient knowledge of many activities so as to be an intelligent spectator and to be able to carry his share of the conversation when such sports events are being discussed.
10. There is little necessity for the average person to know anything about first aid for common injuries suffered in sports because there is always an expert on hand to take care of accidents.

These statements will serve to illustrate the type of material that can be covered with knowledge tests. Teachers will undoubtedly wish to make up their own tests upon the material they have covered in classes or have assigned to students.[16] Such tests, properly used, will indicate areas of student need, will serve as valuable educative and discussion material, and will be of considerable use in determining a part of each student's mark.

The use of other types of records and data for determining student needs

In addition to the technics discussed thus far, the physical educator should make considerable use of other data derived

16 See: Voltmer, E. F. and Esslinger, A. A. *The Organization and Administration of Physical Education,* Chapter 18. Crofts and Co., New York, 1938.
   See also: Staley, S. C. and Stafford, G. T. *A Sports Curriculum.* The Stipes Publishing Co., Champaign, Ill., 1938. Gives illustrations of materials covered in knowledge tests in the University of Illinois service program for men.
   Also: Chapter VI of this study, pp. 90 and 99.

from records in the dean's office, from the office of the guidance and personnel department, or from other sources. The student's I. Q. rating will be of some significance, although the type of intelligence that is usually measured by intelligence tests is not indicative of what the student is able to learn in physical education. The results of aptitude tests, character and personality ratings, and so forth should be included on the student's physical education personal record card. The more measures the educator has of the individuals with whom he is working, the better all-round picture he will have of them. This will aid him to interpret better the data derived through the use of the technics indicated in this chapter. In this way student needs will be discovered and a program which seems to fit the needs of a student can be laid out. This matter of determining needs is a never-ending process. It is wise to give knowledge tests periodically to ascertain if the desired results are being obtained. The use of other technics, such as rating scales, should be employed at frequent intervals for checking or discovering needs.

Summary

By gaining the student's confidence and cooperation, the physical educator can use as educative devices such technics as the health examination, cumulative record card, survey, rating scales, knowledge tests. Students must be encouraged to face the facts which the data from the record reveal, to work out a program for college days and for adulthood in keeping with these facts, and to consider the service program as a phase of education which makes it possible for them to do these things. The approach of the teacher must always be a positive one—one in which he says: This is the situation. Let's see what you (the student) and I can work out that will be of real and lasting benefit to you. Whenever it appears desirable, the student should be allowed to elect those activities in which he is most interested. On the other hand, if the record of past experiences shows that the student has had sufficient contact with a given activity, he should be guided in the choice of another which fits in with his pattern of needs.

CHAPTER III

A Further Statement of Students' Needs

THE content and method of the course of study for the physical education service program must be chosen and conducted primarily to serve the needs of students. In previous chapters it has been shown that these needs can be determined by the use of investigations, studies, and technics, such as the following:

1. A study and interpretation of the accepted principles of physical education derived from studies of the nature of man: his development, physically, socially, and psychologically.

2. An analysis of tried and tested objectives of physical education as these have been expressed by leaders of this field of education and have been used to demonstrate their value as statements of the purposes of this area of education.

3. A determination of the past experiences of students in the field of physical education and physical recreation in order to assign students to new and valuable activity situations and not to permit them to repeat activities already well learned.

4. A study of facilities and activities sponsored by various recreation organizations within the surrounding community which afford opportunity to continue physical education pursuits in after-school, vacation, and later adult period.

5. The health examination which determines the physical-organic status of each individual at a given time.

6. A study of the recreation interests of students, graduates of educational institutions, and cross sections of the general public's recreation interests within the locality served by the institution.

7. The use of various technics commonly employed by guidance and personnel departments to determine the status of individuals. These technics include interviews, observations, data

from other departments of the school, especially the health and guidance departments, the use of rating scales, record forms, and other devices to determine and record needs of students.

8. Knowledge and information tests which cover the materials taught in the physical education service program.

Some of the needs of students which can be met in the physical education service program are discussed here. This statement of needs is, of necessity, a partial one. As explained in the previous chapter, the needs of a given student can be determined only after technics have been applied and an analysis of the resulting data has been made by both the teacher and the student. This is a never-ending process. Students change and different emphases arise in regard to educational pursuits, which make frequent reappraisals advisable. However, through practical experience in service programs, by means of study and research, and through an analysis of modern statements of the purposes of physical education, the following list of student needs has been drawn up. It is readily discernible that many of these needs cannot be met through an activity program alone. In succeeding chapters a plan of administrative organization, whereby such needs can be adequately supplied by the activity program and by several phases of a supplementary program, will be considered.

Students need to assure the proper development and maintenance of the organic systems of the body.

This has long been a major objective of physical education. It expresses a general need of all students. As Williams states: "All that there is of development, aside from heredity, comes through physical education." [1]

Hetherington,[2] interested in the amount of time that should be devoted to big-muscle activity in order to assure the normal development and maintenance of the organic systems of the body, concluded that at the age of nine a minimum of six hours per day should be devoted to big-muscle activity. This should be

---

[1] Williams, J. F. *Op. cit.*, 1938, p. 270.
[2] Hetherington, Clark. *The School Program in Physical Education.* World Book Co., Yonkers, N. Y., 1922.

decreased gradually with age until it reaches two hours daily for a youth of nineteen.

Wood and Cassidy[3] advocate that for college students at least one and one-half hours per day of big-muscle activity are essential, and for adults at least one hour per day. In each case, the figures are subject to modification for individual cases. But it appears that sufficient time and participation in the correct type of activities to assure this normal organic development are essential in order to meet this need of all students. These are the responsibilities of the department of physical education.

Now the question arises, Can a period of one to two hours daily be devoted to physical education by college students? Under present organization this is doubtful. But the need is there. It must not be overlooked. It is at this point that related needs come into the picture. So it is suggested that students be encouraged to learn both individual and group activities well enough and to receive enough pleasure and satisfaction from them to insure their continuation as recreational sports. During their stay in school the intramural and recreational programs will afford opportunities for continued use and further development of the skills, knowledge, and appreciation that have been acquired in the service program. The phenomenal rise of community recreation facilities and activities indicates that these opportunities will also exist after the college years. But to assure that students will understand the need for continued participation in activities another need must be met.

Each student needs to become reliably informed concerning his own physical-organic status and to know the relationship that physical education bears toward the development and maintenance of this status.

Students not only need opportunities for activity in the service program, but should also possess a *knowledge of the process* through which normal physical-organic development comes about and how it can be maintained. In other words, a mere

[3] Wood, T. D. and Cassidy, R. *The New Physical Education,* p. 67. The Macmillan Co., New York, 1931.

provision by administrators for activity situations is not enough. Students themselves must become aware of the significance of activity for the development of organic vigor. They should know that sound organic vitality is the basis of health, and that it can be achieved and kept only by means of wholesome physical activity throughout life. It is proposed here that knowledge of this sort be pointed out to students in physical education activities and not solely in the hygiene and physiology sections which seem so totally divorced from the activities of the service program. Such knowledge will encourage students to *appreciate* the place of physical education in their lives. The fact that "second wind" is a circulatory phenomenon and that the "warm up" before athletic contests is related to the process of getting one's second wind is knowledge that every college student should have.[4] Students with impaired organic vitality should understand the causes of this condition and be aware of a plan through which they can approach normal. Matters of this kind should be discussed with all students. These represent true physical *education* opportunities and an area of need for all students.[5]

Each student needs to be aided in the development of a philosophy of life which will assure a proper appreciation for wholesome physical recreation in his life's plan.

It is the purpose of education to aid students to become self-directing and to be able to assume the responsibility of shaping a plan of life for themselves. The well-rounded, healthy, responsible, self-adjusted, physically educated individual should learn to look upon participation in physical activity as a life need, to accept it as worth while in itself, and to carry over the spirit of play into work and life.[6] Each student should be encouraged to

[4] For a simple, straightforward discussion of these phenomena see Hall, Bowman. "Training for Middle Distance Runners." *The Scholastic Coach*, March, 1938, p. 8.
Also see: Goldberg, Sam. "Organic Development Explained for High School Track Teams." *The Athletic Journal*, May, 1937, p. 24.
[5] See Chapter V for a more complete discussion of this type of material in the service program.
[6] See: Mitchell, E. D. and Mason, B. S. *The Theory of Play*, Chapter IV, p. 99. A. S. Barnes and Co., New York, 1937, for an elaboration of this point of view.

state his own individual aim of physical education. As he progresses in the acquisition of play skills, knowledge, and appreciations this aim should be restated. It might, however, be something like this:

Each student should aim to seek a knowledge and mastery of the skills, backgrounds, purposes, and values of physical education and to determine their significance to him as an individual in order that he may better appreciate the desirability for life participation in those activities which are physically wholesome, mentally stimulating and satisfying, and socially sound for him.[7]

In American democracy the educated person needs to learn to work and to play with others.[8]

The physical education service program can definitely contribute to this need of students. It is rich in situations in which the rules of sportsmanship can be learned and practiced. Competitive games in the service program cannot be conducted without the highest type of cooperation between team mates, opponents, officials, and in accordance with the rules and regulations of the game. The acceptance of impersonal disciplines, which each student must learn, is essential before such competitive-cooperation is possible. The conduct of each individual is subject to the approval of the group. Standards of behavior are put into actual practice in highly emotional situations. The group shapes the behavior of the individual, yet the individual is respected for what he can contribute to the group. The individual ceases to become an individual. He has responsibilities that are bigger than himself and has the opportunity of losing himself for the good of the cause. He is really learning to work and to play with others. He is learning things that apply to life itself, as Link suggests in the following statement:

"I visualize a civilization which recognizes the potentialities of the individual . . . in such a civilization sportsmanship will not be confined to the athletic field but will be embodied in every phase

---

[7] Adapted from Williams, J. F. *Op. cit.*, 1938, p. 300.

[8] The Educational Policies Commission. *Op. cit.*, p. 77. This is one of the major purposes outlined therein. Quoted with permission of the publisher.

of life, the classroom, the family, the community, the nation. This civilization will make competitive sports the very foundation of its educational system, because here the lessons of sportsmanship, of impersonal disciplines, of social cooperation, of energetic competition . . . are so effectively learned." [9]

Link goes on to make the point that these qualities which can be derived through participation in competitive sports are the basic qualities of personality.

The development of the qualities just enumerated must be taken into consideration in the content and method of the service program. At present, individual sports are assuming great importance because they have a higher degree of carry-over value than most team games. (See Table II, p. 16.) It must not be forgotten, though, that team games are replete with learning opportunities which favor the positive development of sportsmanship and personality. Once out of college the majority of students will no longer have an opportunity for participation in team games. This need must be met in the service program. A balance of team and individual activities is recommended for the service program.

All students need the ability to handle the body in a well-coordinated manner.

This is a need of all students which is important for several reasons:

1. It enables the individual to express himself better through the use of the human body as an instrument of self-expression.

2. It is important in connection with the development of safety skills and the handling of the body in the event of emergencies.

3. It is the source of that pleasure and satisfaction which must accompany physical activity if one is to take sufficient pleasure in activities to continue them in adult life.

4. It results in social approval, which is so important to the individual.

[9] Link, Henry C. *The Re-discovery of Man*, p. 188. The Macmillan Co., New York, 1938. Quoted with the permission of the publisher.

The physical development, reaction time, stature, height, weight, age, and other factors are determinants of the degree of coordination possible for any given individual. Good neuro-muscular coordination can be defined only in terms of each individual student. But each individual student has a need to develop, for himself, a high degree of such coordination.

Students need to have an understanding of correct body mechanics and to know what is "good form" in performance of the natural movements which are the basis of the fundamental skills used in daily life.

These are generally considered fundamental movements:

Walking	Carrying
Running	Striking
Throwing	Swinging
Jumping	Dancing
Catching	Climbing
Lifting	Pushing
Creeping	Pulling
Dodging	

Many of these movements are used in daily life. Few students have ever had the correct form of walking illustrated to them. The performance of such everyday skills as opening windows, lifting heavy objects, carrying weights, etc., has rarely been discussed as a form of physical education. Yet skills such as these have been advocated for some time by experts in the field, as coming within the realm of the physical education program.[10] Students have need for such instruction. It takes little time, can be made very interesting in class discussions, and affords information that will be of value for all time.

There are many principles of physical education in this area of body mechanics.[11] It will contribute toward meeting the needs

[10] Mitchell, E. D. and Mason, B. S. *The Theory of Play,* p. 103. A. S. Barnes and Co., New York, 1937.
See: Williams, J. F. *Principles of Physical Education,* pp. 278 and 320. W. B. Saunders Co., Philadelphia, 1938.
[11] Williams, J. F. *Op. cit.,* p. 320. Also: Williams, J. F., Dambach, J., and Schwendener, N. *Methods in Physical Education,* p. 23. W. B. Saunders Co., Philadelphia, 1933.

of students to bring these principles and their application before them. The discussions need be neither highly professional nor dry and uninteresting. Students do have an interest in body mechanics, and a desire to improve their performance of the fundamental movements. By using actual illustrations of daily tasks which require these movements and by comparing the way several students do them, real learning situations can be established by the skilled teacher.

Students need to become well qualified as participants and as spectators in many sports.

Here is a need of students which is expressed as one of the major purposes of education.[12] This is a statement, not of one, but of many closely related needs. To become well qualified as a participant in *many* sports means that the service program must afford opportunities for students to learn about many sports by doing. Such sports must be selected that will be of value to students now and in the future. A balance of team and individual sports has already been recommended. Physically educated persons must be not only participants but spectators as well. This implies that students, in order to be appreciative and intelligent spectators, must be aware of:

1. Correct form in the various fundamentals of many activities in order that they may recognize excellence when they see it.

2. The rules, regulations, and "ground rules" of many sports in order that they may intelligently follow the game.

3. The strategy of the game in order that they may experience the thrill of "quarterbacking" or anticipating what the individual or team is to do next.

4. Good manners or the code of ethics acceptable for spectators of the contest. A knowledge of spectator etiquette. For instance, traditionally, different standards of conduct have arisen for different activities. The spectator of a golf match is expected to observe the rule of "Quiet, Please." The spectator of a baseball game is governed by a different code of ethics. Ten-

[12] Educational Policies Commission. *The Purposes of Education in American Democracy*, pp. 50 and 63. Washington, D. C., 1938.

nis also has its specific code of spectator behavior, as do other types of activities.

The physically educated person should be aware of conduct becoming an intelligent, appreciative, educated spectator. Through actual participation in many sports, a keener appreciation of good conduct for spectatorship should be gained. Definitely organized lecture, discussion, illustration periods will assure that sufficient emphasis is being placed upon this phase of physical education.[13] It is a significant area of student need. A few standards of behavior will be listed here. Others will occur to teachers of the various activities of the program.

1. Be quiet when others are teeing off, addressing a ball, or putting at any time on a golf course.

2. Do not wear high-heeled shoes on a golf course.

3. Always applaud excellence on the part of a player of your team or an opponent.

4. Remember that the home team's captain is responsible for the behavior of spectators and may be penalized for unacceptable behavior on their part.

5. Know that the conduct of a sports spectator is governed by traditions of behavior. For example, the "Quiet, Please" of golf does not apply to football or baseball, except in particular instances.

6. Keep in mind that "just good manners" is a reliable guide to one's behavior at an athletic contest.

7. Be considerate of persons adjoining you in the stands.

8. Keep out of established runs unless actually using them in relation to snow sports. Never walk in a ski trail because foot tracks will make it rough, hazardous, and slow it up.

9. Always applaud, never boo, an injured man of the opposing team as he leaves the field or floor.

10. Never cheer when a member of the opposing team is penalized.

11. Observe strict silence when a free throw is being attempted in basketball.

12. Do not boo officials' decisions.

[13] See: Chapters V and VI.

The following excerpt from a daily sports page indicates the need for instruction in spectator behavior:

6000 Collegiate Voices "SH-H-H-H" As One Loud Man[14]
"It is not too late to record a recent prank of (a) rooting section, which must be seen and heard to be believed.

"When the . . . Cagers clashed a week ago, the (home) rooters got into the swing of things and booed lustily every time (an opponent) stepped up to the free throw line. That was on Friday night.

"Before Saturday night's game started (the Yell-leader) took over the loud speaker and asked that the rooters, in the name of common courtesy, refrain from booing (opponents) on the free throw line. (The) request, quite naturally, was greeted with boos.

"The game hadn't gone a minute before (the opponent's) star forward was fouled. As he stepped up to shoot his charity toss every undergraduate in the joint let loose with an explosive "Shhhhhh" which nearly tore the roof off. It sounded as though 11,000 cobras had been turned loose.

"(Note—he missed the free throw.)"

Sharman [15] states that we in physical education must definitely plan our teaching so as to develop a knowledge and appreciation of the fine points of American sports for *all* students. He suggests the following ways by which this can be done:

1. The use of motion pictures.

2. Explanations at school assemblies.

3. Explanations by officials or well-qualified announcers during interruptions of games.

4. Promotion of an extensive intramural program.

5. Definite teaching toward this end in the required physical education classes.

6. The preparation and distribution of a "primer in football" and similar manuals of appreciation for other sports.

7. Provision of games during the regular school hours with all pupils attending and officials lecturing on the fine points of the game.

14 Dick Friendlich in the *San Francisco Chronicle,* February 25, 1940. Quoted with permission of the publisher.

15 From: *Modern Principles of Physical Education,* p. 88, by Jackson R. Sharman. Copyright, 1935, by A. S. Barnes and Co., Inc. Quoted with permission of the publisher.

The point of view taken here is that definite teaching in the service program should be the means of acquainting students with the fine points of games they will be called upon to see, and that a definite emphasis should be laid upon behavior expected of the physically educated spectator at such games. Such knowledge and appreciations are considered here as needs of all students. It is the responsibility of the service program in physical education to meet these needs.

Students need to learn to judge success and failure in physical education pursuits in relation to their own individual capacities.

Many students become discouraged because they cannot meet an "athletic standard" of performance in activities. While they should constantly strive to raise their levels of performances, they should be led to understand that excellence is relative, depending upon many factors—physical coordination, painstaking practice over a long period of time, endurance, strength, body build, reaction time, etc. All students cannot expect to reach a level of excellence comparable to that of a Sammy Snead, a Johnnie Weismuller, or a Donald Budge.

Keep Your Eye On The Ball

Consider the game of golf and its teacher, the club professional. I go, an ignorant tyro, to the course with a friend and am determined to learn the game so that I can hold up my head without shame among my fellows. With a wise companion, or a canny professional, I start on my way to mediocrity and happiness. Mediocrity is success. I know my handicap, and so does every one of my partners. I improve my drive until not many balls are sliced over the fence; I master the niblick so that I can get out of the sand in one, or two, or three strokes; I average only a little over two putts to the green. Also I learn the courtesies and traditions of the game, revel in the companionship it brings, envy the style of the club champion, but never expect to achieve it, and of course bow in adulation with all the others before the Joneses, the Hagens, and the Littles.

The game is a part of life; at times it is life. I am content to remain in mediocrity, for the game is built, is played, is enjoyed, is supported, by mediocrities like myself. I appreciate and admire the expert. But more satisfying to my soul is my own straight hundred and eighty yarder, or my own fifteen foot putt, than all the exploits of the national champions. I must be a producer, a worker, a participant in golf or I would forsake it. So would the rest of the Saturday afternoon foursome.[16]

The point of view illustrated in this article should be acquired by all persons who participate in sports, once they have brought their level of performance to a creditable point. With this point of view students will no longer be reluctant to take part in activities even though their performance is not of championship caliber. They need to appraise their own abilities in this area of education and to set standards accordingly. In lectures and discussions, and upon the play field students should be encouraged to develop pride in performance that is in keeping with their own abilities.

Individuals need to learn how to exercise safety precautions in connection with the performance of physical skills.

It has been mentioned that the development of neuro-muscular skills and of bodily coordination is, in a sense, a form of safety education. That is, ease of handling the body in physical skills will frequently prevent accidents in hazardous games and contests. This ability will also, in a general way, equip one to judge the size and rate of speed of moving objects which might inflict injury upon contact. A fast, controlled response of the body when it is necessary to run and jump from or dodge moving objects is also a form of safety education which is acquired and improved upon by participation in activities which develop neuro-muscular skills and bodily coordination. But there are other factors to be considered in regard to safety in the performance of physical skills.

There is great emphasis, particularly at the present time, upon safety education. The practice of making games and contests as safe as possible for participants and spectators has always been a major administrative problem in physical education. It is not only an administrative objective, however, but also an obligation of each individual who takes part in the program. Students should be trained to recognize possible safety hazards, such as

16 R. F. Bown, in "Alpha Beta Newsletter," October, 1935.

faulty equipment, the throwing of hard or heavy objects in the presence of an uncontrolled crowd, the proximity of benches, trees, etc., to play areas, inadequate landing surfaces for jumping, tumbling, or hazardous gymnastics, and other common hazards that exist in connection with activities.

Physical educators should discuss safety education with the students in the service program in general terms and in relation to each of the activities performed. The relationships of the playing rules to safety should be pointed out. An object lesson should be made of every avoidable accident that occurs in the administration of the service program. Each student should be made personally responsible for avoiding accidents.

Practical knowledge of first aid should also be a part of the equipment of the physically educated person. While this work is done by the proper authorities in school, it must be remembered that it is the obligation of the service program to prepare students for life participation in physical activity—much of which is somewhat hazardous. In these life situations it is not always possible for the injured person to turn to a nurse or physical educator for first aid treatment. He will probably have to do it himself. A knowledge of the rudiments of first aid therefore is a student need. Instruction in this important phase of physical education can be carried on in connection with the various activities of the program, or as a part of an "introductions course," or in a separate first aid course.[17]

One division within the service program is aquatics. It is a very important division because of its great carry-over value. Each student ought to know how to save his own or another's life in the water. Lifesaving technics and resuscitation should be known to all students. Much of present-day recreation is centered at the seashore, the lakes, the rivers, and the streams of the nation. The service program can educate students for emergencies in these recreational pursuits which are a part of the lives of so many people.[18]

[17] See: Chapter V.
[18] The latest material on first aid, swimming and diving, and lifesaving may be secured from local representatives of the American Red Cross.

Students need an understanding of how games and activities can be modified to be carried on in limited areas, with makeshift equipment, and with larger or smaller numbers of people than the official rules designate.

The physically educated person must not be denied play opportunities merely because of limitations of supplies, play space, or numbers of people. Most of the activities that are included in the service program can be so modified that students will never lack opportunities to take part in them. "Picnic Baseball" is an example. Because of small area, rough ground, lack of official bases, varying numbers of people, and other factors it has been the usual custom to modify the "National Game" so that it could be a part of the recreation program of outings. For this purpose softball is recommended instead of hardball. The fourteen-inch ball does not go as far as the standard twelve-inch ball. Bats can be so modified that they do not have the striking power of the standard bat. Base lines can be shortened if the area is small or the age of the players indicates that it would be wise to do so. Similarly, the distance of the pitcher from the plate can be lengthened. If smaller numbers of people wish to play, the size of the diamond can be made smaller, that is, instead of the usual 90 degree angle at the home plate a 60 degree angle can be drawn. It is also possible to eliminate second base in this smaller diamond. With still smaller numbers of people the traditional "One Old Cat" will enable the game to go on. A variation of "One Old Cat," in which several persons who are at bat must start at right field and again "work up" once they are put out, is familiar to most persons.

Basketball played at only one basket with a soccer ball or a volleyball, when a basketball is not available, is a good game for recreational purposes.

There are any number of games of "Golf" which can be adapted for use in the parlor, a small back lot, the front lawn, and

---

See: Eastwood, Floyd R. "Causes of College Sport Accidents." *The Research Quarterly,* October, 1934.

Also: Lloyd, F. S., Deaver, G. G., and Eastwood, F. R. *Safety in Athletics.* W. B. Saunders Co., Philadelphia, 1936.

other areas. The soft golf balls obtainable at sporting goods dealers make it possible to work on "The Swing" indoors without danger.

Soft, woolly balls are now available for badminton. These make the game more economical and also make it possible to play it in smaller areas than the standard court size.

The practice of handicapping will also suggest ways in which players of unequal ability can adapt games so that the contest may go on. Students should be familiar with the purposes and means of handicapping.[19]

Many team, as well as individual, activities can be modified by simple changes of rules, of playing equipment, and of play areas in such a way that they can be enjoyed when opportunities are not available for "official contests." The criticism is often made that the games in physical education are conducted under ideal conditions which are seldom approximated in life participation. Unless college physical education is merely a recreational program to be participated in by students only while they are in school, it will be of benefit to them to show how games can be modified. Discussion groups, in which students are asked to volunteer examples of how to modify various activities, or in which they report modifications they have seen, will prove interesting to students and instructors alike.[20]

Students need to become proficient in activities in which they may participate with members of the opposite sex.

In recent years there has been considerable emphasis upon the inclusion of coeducational activities within physical education programs. If physical education activities are to make up a part of the lives of educated persons, it follows that some attention must be given in the service program to activities which are suitable for both men and women to participate in at the same time. Yet there are a number of factors that must first be considered. It is generally agreed that games with considerable bodily contact

[19] Williams, J. F. and Morrison, W. R. *A Textbook of Physical Education,* p. 303. W. B. Saunders Co., Philadelphia, 1939.
[20] See: Chapter VI, pp. 90 and 101.

are not suitable for this purpose. Neither is it desirable to play games in which the members of one sex must "let down" in order to equalize play. This soon kills the "play spirit" of both. It appears that games with the following characteristics are best suited to coeducational situations:

1. There should be no rough bodily contact possible.
2. Strength and high degrees of endurance should not be primary elements of the games.
3. Activities in which the principal element is skill are desirable.
4. Activities which can be equalized by means of handicapping, as in golf, are desirable.

These criteria suggest that the following activities are excellent for coeducational participation:

Golf	Hiking	Archery	Shuffleboard
Tennis	Riding	Camping	Social dancing
Badminton	Fishing	Boating	Tap dancing
Swimming	Hunting	Ping Pong	Bowling

More emphasis should be placed upon these activities in the service program. Some of the instruction periods can well be organized so that both sexes may be present. Coeducational classes in golf, social dancing, archery, badminton, riding, shuffleboard, ping pong, and similar activities are now a part of the course of study in a number of colleges and universities. This trend is wholesome and in keeping with modern purposes of education. It makes possible opportunities which will better enable students to adjust themselves to members of the opposite sex. It provides opportunities for the development of personality as well as sex adjustment.

If the service program is to contribute to this need of students for coeducational participation in physical recreation pursuits, it must be conducted according to the principle of "learning by doing." Wherever possible, coeducational classes in activities that meet these criteria are recommended for the service program in physical education.

Students need an understanding of the cultural heritage and development of the well-known sports of America, the place they have in the service program, and the place they occupy in the everyday lives of American citizens.

The physically educated person needs to have an understanding and appreciation of the sports of America. For instance, he should know that baseball is considered America's national game in spite of the fact that it was originally a combination of the English games of rounders and cricket.[21] He should also know that basketball and volleyball are games that are truly American in origin. The history and development of American football, of golf, of track and field events, and of other sports should be known to all educated Americans. Such knowledge can be made available to students in a number of ways. As each of these activities is taken up in the service program a short period of time can well be devoted to lectures, discussions, and illustrations regarding the origin, history, and development of each activity.[22] The reason why some sports have developed and have been accepted by the people of America should be discussed. The class should be called upon to determine why its members like some games and not others. Another way in which this material can be made available is by means of classroom sections. These sections can be definitely organized and scheduled, or can take place as "rainy day" sections.[23] In such sections the students become aware of the origin, history, and development of the sports of America, discuss reasons for their popularity in relation to the social psychology of America—in short, add to their knowledge and appreciation of facts that should be commonly known to the educated person.

[21] See: Menke, Frank G. *The All Sports Record Book*. 235 East 45 St., New York, N. Y. Published annually. Includes origin, history, records, and highlights of all sports.

Also: Mitchell, E. D. (edr.) *Sports for Recreation*. A. S. Barnes and Co., New York, 1936.

[22] See: Chapter VI.

[23] See: Chapter V.

In a democracy, students need to learn to lead and to follow as well as to recognize in which of the two capacities they may best serve the group cause.

There appear to be two types of leadership which can be developed in physical education situations. The first is exemplified by the individual who excels or rates high in some field of human endeavor so he may be called a leader in that field. A Bobby Jones, a Donald Budge, or a Glenn Cunningham, performers who excel in a given activity to the point where they become a source of inspiration and example to many people, are exemplary of individuals displaying this type of leadership.

The second type of leadership is illustrated by one such as a team captain, who commands the respect of his fellows not only because of ability as a performer but also because of the following traits:

1. He is able to recognize a situation which presents an opportunity for leadership.

2. He can see the problems involved in the situation.

3. He can see a solution, or a plan of action for the solution of the problems.

4. He has the personal qualities for leadership.

Physical education pursuits, properly conducted, have great potentialities for the development of leadership. As one source points out:

Few, if any, school subjects provide the number of leadership opportunities that are to be found in physical education. It provides a more complete means of educating *through* physical education since it permits the students to share in the various aspects of leadership which the instructor directs.[24]

The service program in physical education is replete with opportunities for the emergence of leadership. Team games, in particular, require and develop leaders. Leadership emerges

[24] Voltmer, E. F. and Esslinger, A. A. *The Organization and Administration of Physical Education,* p. 291. F. S. Crofts Co., New York, 1928. Quoted with permission of the publisher.

when a group or team is working toward a common goal. Leadership is closely akin to cooperativeness. Without a high degree of cooperativeness a team would be unable to function. In the schools of a democracy successful cooperation should be a part of the experience of all students.[25]

The physical educator should recognize leadership, encourage its development, and provide situations in which students can increasingly rise to positions of higher responsibility. This can be done by appointing and rotating captains in the team games' part of the program, and by encouraging student representatives to aid in drawing up schedules, regulations, and procedures of competition. Leadership can be fostered by allowing students with outstanding qualities to act as organizers and officials, if such duties do not interfere with their opportunities to represent their teams.

Students need opportunities in which to "forget themselves" for the time, in order that they can have opportunities to re-create themselves.

Physical education, in American schools, was originally sponsored because of the values that were associated with it as a remedial agency. Its purpose then was to alleviate the monotony and staleness of the academic program.[26] It is not proposed here that this is the sole purpose of physical education. But it must not be forgotten that we now live in an age of stress, cares, worries, and pressures of many kinds. The academic program in many schools has the effect of pressure upon students while they are in school. The cares and worries one experiences upon completion of school days in connection with one's life work are also likely to be numerous and heavy. Both in-school and out-of-school physical education can serve importantly to provide opportunities in which students "forget themselves" for the time being. A hotly contested handball game, a round of golf, or a few sets of tennis in the company of persons of equal skill, accompanied with

[25] See: The Educational Policies Commission. *The Purposes of Education in American Democracy*, p. 78. Washington, D. C., 1938.
Also: Voltmer, E. F. and Esslinger, A. A. *Op. cit.*, Chapter XI.
[26] See: Williams, J. F. *Op. cit.*, 1938, p. 215.

congeniality and good-natured badinage do much to re-create a person.

An individual's ability and desire to take part in activities is dependent, it is true, upon the skills, attitudes, and appreciations he has developed and accepted in regard to physical education activities. The development of these skills, attitudes, and appreciations has also been considered a student need which can be served in the service program. Students require preparation to the point where they can "forget themselves" for the time.

Students need to be able to recognize and analyze the claims of fakers, quacks, and physical cultists regarding physical education.

There are still many individuals who are attempting to exploit the natural desire of the young people of America to have a strong, healthy, well-proportioned physique. Deep breathing exercises are counted out over the morning radio, as are complicated calisthenics for the avowed purpose of "physical conditioning." Certain periodicals of wide circulation offer "short courses" of calisthenics and body building exercises which, it is claimed, will result in strong, virile manhood for the individual who will send a fee and faithfully practice the exercises sent to him.

College physical education can provide opportunities wherein students learn to analyze the claims of physical cultists. These claims can be examined and criticized in the light of the true structure and function of the human body. The analysis can be taken a step further to show the relationship of structure and function to physical exercise and health. For example, it is a well-known fact that as the body requires more oxygen for increased work, the respiratory rate will automatically increase in both rate and degree. Deep breathing exercises have no scientific justification. Indeed, if they are persisted in they can bring about a condition of dizziness and can even cause fainting. This is nature's way of indicating that they are harmful. In the discussion of the health examination it was pointed out that complicated, sustained movements of arms, legs, and torso, without regard for the physical condition and needs of each unique individual, might likewise prove harmful.

Suppleness, coordination, and grace of movement are goals of modern physical education. A maximum "culture" or the development of maximum strength of muscle groups of the body is not compatible with modern purposes of physical education. In fact, a condition commonly known as "muscle bound" may be the result of over-development of the muscle groups of the body. The principle of opposition indicates that true symmetry of the human body is not a normal condition. That is, the right-handed person will normally be better developed muscularly in the right arm and shoulder and the left leg, and the right shoulder may be an inch or more lower. This would indicate a perfectly normal condition. Yet, true symmetry of the body is one of the goals of "physical cultists."

Students have a need for knowledge based upon scientific findings concerning the structure and function of the human body. This knowledge is essential in order that they can protect themselves from the claims of unscrupulous persons who are attempting to sell a "system" or equipment that will promote "physical culture." Such knowledge can be afforded students through the physical education service program by means of lectures, discussions, and similar technics. The school physician might be called upon to explain such matters to classes, provided he does so in non-technical terms so that the students will understand the subject matter. In any event, this is an area of student need to which the service program can contribute. If needs such as these are not cared for through the service program, significant educational opportunities will be overlooked. Modern physical education can no longer be merely recreational, it must become educational as well.

Students need to develop consumer judgment, efficiency in buying, and consumer protection in relation to the purchase of sports equipment.[27]

In connection with physical education pursuits in school, as well as physical recreation and sports pursuits out of school, indi-

[27] These are three of the purposes of education outlined by The Educational Policies Commission in *The Purposes of Education in American Democracy*, p. 90. Washington, D. C., 1938. Quoted with permission of the publishers.

viduals purchase considerable sports equipment. The physical education service program can be so conducted that students are educated as consumers of such equipment. They should be able to identify good equipment, recognize what is a fair price, and know how to care for it in order to receive maximum benefit. There is a great variety of sports equipment on the market. Students need standards upon which to make wise selections. For instance, the beginning golfer who is operating on a budget should know that a No. 2 wood (brassie), a No. 2 iron (midiron), a No. 5 iron (mashie), and a putter are sufficient for the novice. He should also know that clubs should be selected from an open pattern so that the set can be added to as he becomes more proficient. He should know what length clubs to buy in relation to his body build.[28] The beginner should also know that a ball with a tough cover is more economical for his purposes than the thinly covered, easily cut, championship ball, even though the latter can be driven a few yards further.

The user of a gut strung racket should know that rackets are of different weights and balances. He should know the importance of keeping the racket in a press when not in use, as well as the fact that a wet court is very injurious to it.

There are thousands of young people in America now interested in the purchase of winter sports equipment. It is estimated that the number of skiers has tripled each year in the past three years in the United States.[29] Winter sports clothing should be warm, light, and waterproof. The old rule of selecting the length of skis according to one's reach no longer holds. Table VI is a much more reliable guide.

The rule usually holds that it is poor economy to buy inferior sports equipment, and that for the average performer it is unnecessary to buy championship equipment. A middle ground should be adapted after a thorough investigation of equipment.

[28] Wood clubs are now sold in two lengths: standard and long; irons in standard and short lengths. Custom built clubs are made to measurement. A person's height and arm length are important factors in the selection of golf clubs.

[29] *Ski Manual for 1940.*

See: Putnam, Harold (edr.). *The Dartmouth Book of Winter Sports.* A. S. Barnes and Co., New York, 1939.

TABLE VI

LENGTH CHART FOR SKIS AND POLES *

Ski Length	Height	Weight	Sex	Pole Length
6'	5' 2"	90 to 120	Children and women	46"
6' 3"	5' 4"	115 to 130	Children and women	48"
6' 6"	5' 6"	125 to 140	Women and men	50"
6' 9"	5' 10"	140 to 165	Women and men	52"
7'	6'	150 to 185	Men	54"

Note: Over 7' lengths recommended for racers only.

* Ski Manual for 1940. Gerber Bros., 2600 First Ave., Seattle, Wash. Quoted with permission of the publishers.

Many further examples of opportunities to aid students in the selection and care of sports equipment might be cited. This information, as illustrated in Table VI, will indicate that consumer efficiency in regard to sports equipment is a need of students which should be met in the service program. Many dispensers of sports equipment will offer the purchaser aid in the selection and care of equipment. As a part of his physical education the student should be guided in the development of standards upon which to make consumer judgments.[30]

Students need to be able to understand the literature of sports and recreation, to know how to read and interpret the sports page, how to watch an athletic contest, and other related information concerning sports and contests that constitute a part of their daily lives.

America is becoming increasingly sports conscious. The material to be found in the daily sports sections of the local newspapers offers topics for discussion at the table, in the club, in the living room—in short, wherever groups of people gather. To be able to listen intelligently, as well as contribute to the conversation, one must have an understanding of the terminology of sports, how to keep score, how to arrange handicaps, and the various types of tournaments (round robin, elimination,

[30] See: Williams, J. F. and Hughes, W. L. *Athletics in Education.* W. B. Saunders Co., Philadelphia, 1936, for a detailed discussion in regard to the purchase and care of athletic equipment.
See: Chapter VI.

match play, medal play, etc.), what is meant by "seeding players," what "par" is in golf and how it is determined, what is meant by such commonly used terms as "stymie," "birdie," "eagle," "Slalom," "Christiana," "zone defense," "interference with the passer," "in" and "out" in golf, etc.

Proficiency in the use of terms should be acquired as a part of the experiences in the physical education service program. As students learn the fundamental skills of activities, so should they learn the terminology to be identified with them, together with the backgrounds, rules, and regulations.[31]

Sports pages and sports articles in current periodicals should be discussed with students. As each activity is introduced into the service program, attention should be paid to the terminology and other aspects of the activity with which one should be thoroughly familiar. These materials should be made a part of regular discussions in physical education.[32]

Such knowledge can be used to form the basis of knowledge tests in each activity, as well as tests regarding rules, regulations, and technics of performance. This approach in physical education contributes to the needs of students and is also a significant factor in the development of appreciations of physical education. In this way students can become intelligent not only about the activities in which they actually participate, but about many other activities that are a part of the daily lives of many of the people of America. This need is closely allied to one previously discussed, namely, to make students intelligent spectators of sports contests.

Summary

This investigation of student needs, although necessarily a general one, indicates that if these needs are to be met in the physical education service program, something more than the traditional recreational-activity sports sections is required. Par-

[31] See: Chapter VI.

[32] For materials in such learning situations see Williams, J. F. and Morrison, W. R. *A Textbook of Physical Education.* W. B. Saunders Co., 1939.

Also: Little, Lou and Harron, R. *How to Watch Football, The Spectator's Guide.* McGraw-Hill Book Co., New York, 1935.

ticularly is this true when general needs are refined into individual needs.

In the following chapters it is indicated that individual needs can be met by means of an advisory system which affords students both individual and group guidance. The traditional activity program is not sufficiently broad to meet all of the needs of students in regard to physical education pursuits. Therefore, several ways in which the program can be supplemented and enriched will be discussed.

CHAPTER IV

The Supplementary Program: Orientation

The need for orientation periods

PREVIOUS statements of student needs indicate that they are both numerous and varied. If needs are to be met in the physical education service program, situations must be provided which will promote several types of learnings. The enriched program should include: (1) An opportunity to perform the fundamental skills, which are encountered daily, in addition to the technics and skills of several team and individual sports, especially those that will be continued in recreational pursuits at the completion of college work. (2) The formulation by each student of a philosophy of physical education which will encourage a lifelong participation in some form of physical education activity. To "play for the sake of play" should be a primary motive. (3) A knowledge and understanding of the origin, backgrounds, and development of sports and contests, and the place of these in our American life today. (4) A knowledge of proper conduct of sportsmanship and etiquette to be displayed either as a participant or as a spectator. (5) A thorough understanding of the significant relationships of physical education to health, to other subject matter fields, to the athletic program, to community recreation, and to the whole range of life activities.

In order to promote learning situations of this broad nature the physical activity program must be supplemented. While physical activity will always be the basic content, related learnings must be encouraged if this area of education is to assume its rightful place in the challenge to meet student needs. Routine physical training in technics and skills does not fill the bill. Williams[1] points out that concomitant learnings accom-

[1] See: Williams, J. F. *Principles of Physical Education*, pp. 376 and 398. W. B. Saunders Co., Philadelphia, 1938.

pany the acquisition of physical skills. It is also true that these
supplementary learnings may be positive and educationally desirable, or negative and undesirable. It is proposed, in view of
the many significant related learnings which must be brought to
the attention of students, that the organization of the physical
education program be very broad and comprehensive. With
the proper emphasis upon the important concomitant learnings,
the physical education program will be more than a training
of muscles.

If there is to be any reasonable surety that students are gaining knowledge and an understanding of relationships to form a
background upon which to base attitudes, interests, and appreciations of physical education, a concrete plan of graded instruction is essential. There appear to be three related ways in which
this can be effected:

1. By means of an "Orientation Period" during which all new
   students become familiar with the organization, administration,
   significance, and relationships of other fields to physical education. This period is usually conducted for all new students
   prior to regular registration and is a form of group guidance to
   acquaint students with the offerings of the institution, its facilities, etc. It is also a period during which various diagnostic
   tests are given.

2. By means of definitely organized classes of "Introductions and
   Appreciations of Physical Education" in which the backgrounds, purposes, and values of physical education are pointed
   out to all students. The appreciations course conducted by the
   physical education staff to give credit as do other courses in the
   general curriculum.

3. By means of instruction units in connection with each of the
   activity sections of the course of study. These units to require
   readings, reports, class notes, and examinations covering technics, rules, etiquette, sportsmanship in addition to the origin,
   development, and trends of each activity.

It appears that each of these plans has definite educational
value. The "Orientation Period" acquaints students with fundamental relationships in a brief overview of what this particular
field of the curriculum is attempting to do to meet their needs.

It is a form of group guidance which, it is hoped, may alleviate many misunderstandings that occur in the subsequent program-making period. The "Introductions and Appreciations" course takes up in some detail the concepts outlined in the "Orientation Period" and also includes instruction in supplementary materials of activities—which should comprise a part of the fund of knowledge of every educated man. The instruction units are confined to the sport or activity with which they are identified. They indicate the level of achievement to be attained, and afford opportunities for students to make use of library materials to supplement the instruction given in the physical skills and technic of the activity. These units include significant information concerning etiquette, sportsmanship, and standards of conduct materials, which too often are overlooked. Carefully constructed tests based on these units permit a more objective means of marking.

These plans are not mutually exclusive. Nor do they involve needless repetition. If properly organized and conducted they richly supplement the activity program and provide opportunities for study which can stand up in the light of the most searching educational scrutiny. Instruction units and the classes in introductions and appreciations of physical education will be discussed in chapters to follow. A plan whereby the orientation period may be organized and conducted will be outlined here.

The orientation period

Many schools now require new students to report to the campus in advance of the regular registration period in order to take diagnostic tests and examinations of various types: intelligence and aptitude tests, and subject "A" examinations in English. During this period, also, the health examination is taken. Advisers are available during this time. The results of the examinations are immediately recorded on file cards and used by advisers in aiding students to select a well-balanced program.

There is a definite need for the physical education department, as one of the important subject matter fields of the curriculum, to organize its part in this general scheme of orientation. There is probably more misunderstanding in regard to the organization of the several divisions of physical education, their purposes and values, and conduct than for any other field of the curriculum. Even though the institution as a whole does not have an orientation period the physical education department will be rendering a significant service to students by providing one. These meetings should be scheduled in advance of the opening of school. They should be well publicized and a schedule of them given to each student as a part of the first step of admittance to the institution. In fact, they should be included in the announcement of courses of the institution.

Content of the orientation period[2]

Each institution will have a characteristic plan of organization for orientation periods. Each physical education department, likewise, will have a particular plan regarding organization and content as it best applies to that institution or department. The following plan is offered as a general suggestion of the type of material that should be included in the orientation period:

I. The head of the physical education department should welcome students and introduce all staff members, including the athletic and health staffs. He should briefly outline points such as the following:

    A. That the requirement is in effect to assure that all students will have opportunities to benefit through participation in some form of physical education.

    B. That the program, for definite purposes, consists of a balance of team and individual activities.

    C. That the program is organized so that students may have interesting and vigorous recreational oportunities while in school and also may learn one or more activities that can be carried over into adult leisure-time recreation.

    D. That the emphasis is placed upon instruction in order that the desired learning shall not be left to chance.

[2] The best qualified person should present each phase of content. It must be remembered that this is to be a very brief overview, and that the course of introductions and appreciations will afford opportunity to follow up the orientation material in greater detail. Personnel suggested here is for purposes of general illustration.

E. That in addition to the technics and skills of each of the activities there are other learnings desirable for the physically educated man to acquire. These are called attitudes, understandings, appreciations, and relationships. Also, that the department is organized to provide definite opportunities for such learnings.

F. That certain relationships exist which guide the physical education staff in the organization and conduct of activities. Relationships of physical education to:
   1. Health and the health department—personal hygiene.
   2. General education—all other areas of the curriculum.
   3. Intramural and intercollegiate athletics.
   4. Community recreation while students and as adults.

G. That the whole process of determining needs and consequent assignment to classes has been established to help students meet needs which are present in this area of life.

H. That as students become better informed they will have greater responsibility in determining their physical education programs.

I. That the close cooperation of each student is essential if the program of meeting student needs is to be effective.

J. That there is necessity for certain regulations to promote safety and sanitation in connection with participation in physical education pursuits.

II. A well-qualified staff member should outline the various offerings of the department, including:

A. A list of all activities.

B. Provisions for beginners and for advanced performers.

C. The proportion of team and individual activities.

D. A brief overview of the purposes of the introductions and appreciations course.

III. A staff member should explain the principal rules and regulations of the department:[3]

A. The requirement (substitutions allowed—if any).

B. The setup of the advisory system in physical education.

[3] See: Chapter VIII.

C. Procedure in case of absence.

D. Credit for physical education.

E. The circumstances under which courses may be repeated for credit.

F. Fees—the amount and uses made of them.

IV. A staff member should explain the location and use of facilities and equipment. This would include:

A. A listing and naming of all facilities, including those used in the athletic program.

B. Community facilities available to students.

C. Rules of conduct pertaining to the use of facilities, including shower and dressing rooms.

D. Physical education uniforms:
  1. How issued.
  2. How exchanged for clean and when.
  3. Procedure in case of loss.
  4. How to care for clothing, the locker or basket system.

V. A member of the athletic coaching staff should explain the following:

A. The relationship of intercollegiate athletics to the service program.

B. The method of coming out for a team.

C. If the school is a member of an athletic conference, the advantages of this membership. (Name other schools in the conference; outline eligibility rules which athletes must meet.)

D. The setup of athletics as controlled by the faculty.

E. Other information which students should have in order to be intelligent regarding the purposes, organization, and conduct of intercollegiate athletics in the institution.

VI. The school physician or a member of his staff should point out:

A. The significance of the health examination and its relationship to physical education, indicating the meaning of the "A," "B," and "C" classifications.

B. The procedure required of students who are re-entering physical education classes after illness or injury or a prolonged leave of absence.

C. The point of view of the medical profession concerning the desirability for life participation in some form of wholesome physical activity.

D. The rules and regulations governing the administration of all phases of health service in the institution.

Upon completion of the above introductory talks, if time permits opportunity should be given for questions. The questions should be directed to each speaker but if the entire staff serves as a panel, the speaker may refer to any member for an answer.

Summary

The orientation period will make it possible for all new students to obtain an overview of the purposes, organization, and conduct of the entire physical education program. If the meetings are carefully planned and the best-qualified staff members are chosen to present the materials, the periods will constitute a significant educational experience. The entire session should be conducted on a level that is understandable to these newcomers. Highly professional and technical materials should be reduced to common terms that are intelligible to students.

A few leading questions by the staff members can do much to stimulate and maintain interest in the procedure. For instance, one might ask: What is physical education? When can we say that one is physically educated? Who determines how many intersectional football games our team may play this year? Are intramurals a feeder for intercollegiate athletics or a supplement to the service program? Why is a health examination required of all students? Questions of this nature usually serve to create interest.

Some of the materials taken up in these first orientation meetings will be explained in more detail in the course of introductions and appreciations by advisers in individual and group conferences, and in the instructional periods for each activity. Material such as that just outlined can be presented in two to four hours, depending, of course, on the amount of detail and the time allowed for questions. Two sessions of two hours each are recommended. In this period of time a great deal can be done to "orient" students regarding the place, purposes, and function of physical education as a phase of the educational curriculum of the institution. As a result, students will be better informed and consequently better prepared to arrive at decisions, with the aid of advisers, regarding their needs and particular phases of physical education which appear best suited for them.

CHAPTER V

The Supplementary Program: Introductions and Appreciations of Physical Education

The traditional activity program and student needs

THE traditional service program for all students, while offering opportunities to learn certain game skills and technics, has failed to realize its inherent potentialities in providing activities whereby students can become physically educated in a broad sense.

One has but to ask a single question of individuals who have passed through the traditional programs, or of students now registered in such a program, to find that the emphasis has been upon physical *training* to the neglect of significant *educational* experiences which rightfully belong in this phase of the curriculum. The true significance of physical education and physical recreation as a phase of the curriculum should be well known by college graduates. A large part of life pursuits are to be identified with physical recreations, either as a participant or as a spectator. The backgrounds, purposes, and values of each of the activities of the program should likewise be known to the physically educated person.

The question is: What is physical education? It will lead to others: Of what value is it to you? How may it become of more value? Are its values confined to school years alone or is it possible to learn skills and information which will enable you to "live most and serve best"? What particular needs do you have which physical education can help you meet? Is there a justifiable place for physical education in the curriculum of educational institutions?

All too frequently students do not have adequate information with which to formulate an objective answer to these queries. The activity program has missed the mark! It has failed to educate adequately through the medium of physical activity. Therefore, the traditional activity program must be supplemented if truly educational experiences, in a broad sense, are to be provided. Half-truths, misinformation, superstitions, and traditional beliefs with no authenticity whatever abound in the conversations of the layman regarding the purposes and values of physical education pursuits. A functional point of view of education insists that students be educated in order that they may be able to judge traditional customs and hand-me-down information in the light of accepted principles of physical education. Yet, most students upon graduation from the usual physical education program cannot define a principle in this field of life preparation. They are, consequently, easy prey for the commercial faker and quack who extols the virtues of a "short course in health, strength, and strong vigorous manhood" by means of a "system of muscular exercises."

Conversations in the street, at the club, in the living room, and elsewhere in daily life are concerned with health, sports, and recreation. Comments like these are heard: Are the breathing exercises and calisthenics broadcast over the morning radio of any value to me? Why do they say 1939 marked the centennial of baseball? How are handicaps arranged in golf? Where can I find the World's Record in the 440? Where did the Olympic Games originate? Of what significance is the Olympic Ideal in relation to contemporary world affairs? What qualifications must the physical education teacher and coach have? Is he an athletic coach or a teacher? Do I walk correctly? Why is basketball called an invented game? Why have track and field records improved so greatly in recent years?

College students are as interested in these questions as the general public. It is functional information they desire. Students have a *need* for such information. Is it too much to say that such knowledge, together with the enriched attitudes and appreciations which inevitably accompany it, is as important as the ability to shoot a basket, master the backswing in golf, or spike a volleyball—all of which can be accomplished with little knowledge of the real purposes underlying such pursuits?

It is proposed here that college physical education, indeed, physical education at all levels, must consider this educational challenge. The present program has an obligation to students which it is not meeting.

Williams explains in great detail the need for including in the physical education curriculum materials other than the physical skills and technics commonly associated with the traditional program:

"It is indeed strange that college students are initiated into the activities of physical education without at any time, until recently, receiving instruction in its backgrounds, its purposes, its results, and its procedures. The freshman who enters college will take other laboratory courses, such as chemistry, physics, geology, and zoology, but the hours in the laboratories of these practices are only a part of an entire course in which the basic content of the subject is presented. Too frequently the student is assigned to a physical education class for activity only; he graduates without even learning anything about the basic content material of physical education. If physical education had no content there might be some excuse for this but its backgrounds are rich and interesting, its results significant, and its procedures helpful when understood. Freshmen in college may be expected to learn, in addition to the practice of the pool, athletic field, and gymnasium, something of the historical background of their laboratory activities, what results may be expected from the practices in which they engage, some common measures of physical education, how learning of motor activities takes place, the laws of training, the use of exercise in training, how to care for oneself in physical education, the principles in movement behind the practice of fundamental motor skills, how to correct certain defects, how to read the sports page of the newspaper, and the proper use of facilities and equipment. The rational basis for credit in physical education is a theory course with laboratory practice. There should be a textbook for the course and all freshmen in college should be given an opportunity to become intelligent about a great area of education.

"Many pressing professional problems in physical education must await an intelligent public opinion. When the average citizen really knows the value of play and understands the contribution of physical education to life, to health, and to happiness, there will be less opposition by boards of education and city officials to greatly extended facilities and personnel for physical education. The distressing problems of professionalism in sport will be met partly by educating the alumni of institutions but this must be done while they are undergraduates. From many points of view there is a real need to help college students to become intelligently informed about physical education." [1]

This opinion forcefully bears out the contention that instruction in physical skills, no matter how excellent, does not constitute an adequate, educationally acceptable physical education program. Significant areas of student needs are not met by a straightforward skill program. In the previous chapter one way of meeting the need—the orientation period—was advocated.

But orientation periods, important as they are, are not sufficient. The backgrounds, purposes, values, and procedures of physical education cannot be adequately handled in a few preliminary meetings. Yet this material must be considered if students are to become sufficiently well informed to make judgments regarding the place of physical education pursuits in their lives as students and adults. Definite organization is needed for the presentation of information which will enable them to see and appreciate the significant relationships between the organization and conduct of physical education in-school and desired outcomes which will be functional in out-of-school life. There appear to be two definite, related areas in which instruction is needed:

1. The physical education field in general. Herein would be stated the relationships to health, education, recreation, and life. The knowledges and understandings which qualify students as *educated* regarding the purposes, values, and procedures of this area of education in preparing for life would be offered.

2. Each of the activities of the physical education program. Instruction in skills and technics, and information regarding the origin, development, and place of the activity in American life,

[1] Williams, J. F. *Principles of Physical Education,* pp. 294–295. W. B. Saunders Company, Philadelphia, 1938. Quoted with permission of the publisher.

necessary in order to be well qualified as participant and as spectator in many team and individual sports, would be offered. Participation in and observation of many sports are definite areas of American life.

In addition to the orientation meetings previously described, there are at least two other ways of supplementing the activity program that will provide enriched opportunities for learning in a broad field of physical education.

1. By means of a definitely organized course of "Introductions and Appreciations of Physical Education" to be required once of all new students.

2. By means of units of instruction supplementary to, and in conjunction with, the teaching of each of the activities of the program. These units would require each student to use library facilities, class notes, and materials obtained through demonstrations, lectures, illustrations, and discussions concerning the origin, development, and trends of the activity in question. Definite attention would also be given to acceptable standards of conduct for the participant and spectator of each of the activities.

Organization of introductions and appreciations course

There are several ways in which such a course can be organized:

1. By including general material of the field of physical education within the instruction units for each of the activities.

It does not appear advisable, however, to combine introductory materials or information leading to an appreciation of the *whole field of physical education and its relationships* with instruction in any single activity of the program. The backgrounds, purposes, values, and procedures of physical education as a phase of the curriculum are sufficiently comprehensive to warrant a definite course. Then, too, as students cannot take very many activities in the short stay in college, they should become acquainted with basic materials of the whole field so as to have a background upon which to base appreciations of physical education and to develop sound interests in play and recreation.

2. By means of a survey course in physical education.

In some schools all new students are assigned to a survey course in physical education for the entire freshman year. These classes usually meet three times a week. Two of these periods are devoted to activity and thus a number of activities are learned in the year's time. The other weekly period is devoted to a lecture-discussion period on the backgrounds and understandings of each of the activities offered and the whole general field of physical education.[2]

The criticism directed at the first plan of organization is also in force here. A confusion may result between the general field of physical education and any one of the activities of the program. Furthermore, the plan does not afford nearly enough time to do justice to each of the activities and the entire field. Then, too, as student needs are considered to be the criteria upon which to assign students to classes, a prescribed course for all students is not recommended unless limitations of staff and facilities make it necessary.[3]

3. The third plan involves the establishment of a regularly organized class or classes of "Introductions and Appreciations of Physical Education" for all new students as a regular required course of the institution.

This course should meet, at the minimum, once a week and carry one point or unit credit toward graduation. This credit may not be substituted for participation and instruction in the physical education activities. This is the recommended plan of organization. It is recognized that long-time planning will be required in many instances before such a course can be included in the curriculum. But physical education is preparation for life, a life that is being lived now as well as in the future. Yet, in most institutions only two units out of a total of one hundred and twenty-four are devoted to preparation for living

---

[2] See: Hughes, W. L. *Administration of Health and Physical Education in Colleges*, Chapter VII. A. S. Barnes and Co., New York, 1935.

Also: McCormick, Hubert J. "Orientation in Physical Education." *The Journal of Health and Physical Education*, March, 1940.

[3] See: Chapter VII, p. 108.

in this area of life. Indeed, a course in introductions and appreciations of physical education should, in a sense, be considered a prerequisite to participation in the activity program. The meager experiences in many secondary school programs make the need for such a course even greater.

THE TEACHER

The success of an introductions and appreciations course is dependent upon the teacher. It must be kept in mind that it is not the purpose of this course to "intellectualize" physical education. There is no place for dead, disconnected "knowledge for the sake of knowledge" in this course. Each meeting of the class should result in a stimulating discussion oriented to the everyday student problems of living in the field of physical education, health, and physical recreation. Teachers and students alike must share the problems which arise. Student discussion is to be encouraged. Experiences in the activity program, assignments to carefully chosen sources, and examinations based upon discussions and readings help to stimulate interest. As the student's background of knowledge and understandings increases, these discussions will grow richer and significant appreciations and attitudes will develop.

In order to conduct such a course the teacher should have a broad outline prepared in advance. This outline is merely for the purpose of assuring that important matters will not be neglected. The teacher should not be unduly concerned if class discussions digress from the prepared outline. The skillful and experienced leader knows that discussion and debate mean that student interest has been achieved. Advantage must be taken of this interest and the class discussions led, not forced, in the directions which, in the superior knowledge and training of the teacher, appear desirable. Experience in conducting such classes soon shows that it is better to ask questions than to lecture. In this way interest is stimulated. Students, in turn, ask questions concerning their own experiences, and as a result of this interchange of questions and discussions, the feeling of being a "part of the course" is developed. Such discussions can readily be guided within the confines of a broad outline by the experienced physical educator.

HOW CONTENT IS DETERMINED

The content of a course of introductions and appreciations of physical education should be determined largely by those student needs which are not adequately met through participation in a program of activities alone. By considering the statement of student needs in Chapter III, by consulting the opinions of experts in the field of health, physical education, and recreation, and by drawing upon a decade of experience in teaching service programs in physical education, including instruction in courses of "Introductions" and "Orientation," the writer has developed the following list of student needs which should be met in an enriched service program. Such a list will be subject to revision as new areas of needs are revealed. Students should have knowledge and understanding in regard to the following:

1. What physical education is: backgrounds, purposes, values.
2. The relationship of physical activity to health.
3. Leisure-time physical recreation pursuits which can be developed in the service program.
4. The status of each as an individual in regard to physical-organic status and the ability to achieve certain levels of performance in sport skills in order that a "self-par" can be established upon which to judge success.
5. Safety precautions in regard to physical pursuits.
6. First aid in connection with injuries commonly associated with participation in physical pursuits.
7. Established principles of physical education based upon objective scientific evidence or best available expert opinion as a background upon which to make judgments regarding the claims of fakers, quacks, and physical cultists.
8. Faulty beliefs commonly accepted by the layman which have no justification when analyzed in terms of principles of physical education.
9. The characteristics of a wholesome co-educational sport.[4]

4 See: Chapter III, pp. 47f.

10. The learning process as it applies to physical education.

11. The laws of training: how to condition oneself for sports participation, how to maintain good condition once it is achieved.

12. A brief, but practical knowledge of the physiology of exercise, as it applies to activities within the student's experience.

13. The field of physical education teaching as a life profession.

14. The organization of the physical education department and the regulations thereof.

15. Relationships of physical education to: intramurals, inter-collegiate athletics, the health department, school and community recreation.

16. The local, regional, state, national, and international organizations that promote sports.

17. The origin, backgrounds, development, and present status of the Olympic Games in relation to the Olympic Ideal.

18. Behavior expected of the educated individual as participant or as spectator of many sports and physical recreations.

19. The conduct of sports matches, including handicapping procedures, terminology connected with the various sports, and sports page material in order to be an intelligent follower of sports.

20. The origin, background, development, present status, and probable trends of many of the sports of America.

Some of the subject matter suggested in this outline naturally will be dealt with very briefly in the orientation periods, some will be included in instruction units in connection with the teaching of each of the sports of the activity program, and some will undoubtedly be acquired by students concomitantly as the activity program is carried on. Much will be considered in the course of introductions and appreciations. This does not mean that there will be unnecessary duplication. Wise planning of the *whole program*—the activities, the units of instruction in each of the activities, the orientation sections, and the course of introductions and appreciations will assure students of a better education in this area of the curriculum.

In preparing an outline for the introductions and appreciations course the teacher must draw upon all of his experiences as a professional student and teacher of health, physical education, and recreation. The actual everyday problems of living in these related fields will largely determine the scope and sequence of the methods and materials of the course. The following outline, together with selected sources, is offered as an example of the type of materials that should be included in such a course.

SUGGESTED CONTENT FOR INTRODUCTIONS AND APPRECIATIONS COURSE *

I. What Physical Education Is.
    A. Historical background. (16)
        1. How physical education came to America. (23:Chap. I)
        2. Systems of physical education, why they have not survived. (26:Chap. VI)
        3. What physical education is in America today. (30:Chap. I) (26:Chap. VIII) (24:Chap. V)
        4. Organizations promoting physical education in America. (1) (27:Chap. I)
    B. Relationships.
        1. Of physical education to:
            a. Health. (25) (26)
            b. Strength. (26:25)
            c. The curriculum as a whole. (7) (8) (11)
            d. Athletics, intramurals and intercollegiates. (28)
            e. Community recreation. (26:Chap. VIII)

II. Principles of Physical Education.
    A. What a principle is. (26:Chap. I)
    B. Why a knowledge of principles is essential in the conduct of physical education practices. (26:Chap. I) (24:1)
    C. Examples of principles based upon: (31:Chap. I)
        1. Anatomy. (26:Chap. III)
        2. Physiology. (26:Chap. III)
        3. Psychology. (26:Chap. IV)
        4. Sociology. (26:Chap. V)
    D. Examples of practices based upon faulty beliefs. (26:25)
        1. Breathing exercises.

* The first number in parentheses refers to the references in the bibliography at the end of this chapter. The second number refers to a page or chapter in the specified reference.

2. Maximum muscular development.
3. That character can be developed through certain types of exercises.
4. That physical education is nothing but exercise.
5. Others.

E. Examples of quackery and exploitation based upon faulty beliefs. (26:Chap. I) (10)
F. Why the physical education programs for men and women have different emphases. (31:Chap. I) (26:84)

III. Physical Education as Education.
A. The unity of man. (26:Chap. IV) (26:266)
B. The fourfold development. (26:Chap. XIII)
   1. Physical-organic. (24:Chap. III)
   2. Neuro-muscular. (26:320)
   3. Psychological. (24:Chap. VI)
   4. Sociological. (24:Chap. V and VII)
C. What the "physically educated individual" is. (26:282)
D. The challenge of this interpretation of physical education to students and educators alike.

IV. Learning in Physical Education.
A. Laws of learnings applied to physical education. (26:Chap. IV and XII) (30:Chap. IV) (24:Chap. VI)

V. Correct "Form" in the Performance of Fundamental Movements Which Are the Basis for All Physical Activity. (26:Chap. X) (30:Chap. VIII)
A. How to:
   1. Walk.
   2. Run.
   3. Jump.
   4. Catch.
   5. Throw.
   6. Strike.
   7. Lift heavy weights.
B. Modifications of fundamental movements for a purpose. (26:322)
   1. The shot put.
   2. High jumping with the "roll" forms.
   3. Swimming.
   4. Skating.
   5. Golf.
   6. Tennis, especially the backhand stroke.
   7. Others.

C. How, for a definite purpose (height, distance, etc.), such modifications represent an improvement upon the "natural way."

VI. The Laws of Training. (30:Chap. V) (29)
   A. The meaning of training. (30:105)
   B. The constant need for training in order to be prepared for a full life and emergencies requiring sudden energy.
   C. Diet. Sleep. Poisons. (30:125–141)
   D. Signs of good and poor condition. (30:146–147)
   E. Second wind. What it is. How it is developed. (30:153) (22:Chap. XV)
   F. Staleness in athletics. What it is. How treated. (30:150) (22:Chap. XVI)
   G. Does participation in heavy athletics injure the heart? (22:Chap. XVIII)

VII. Safety Precautions and First Aid in Connection with Physical Education Pursuits.
   A. Hazardous sports. How to avoid injury. (18)
      1. Preliminary training and conditioning.
      2. Skill in technics minimizes injury.
      3. Physical surroundings must be made safe.
      4. Good judgment must be exercised. Unnecessary chances should be avoided.
   B. First Aid. (4) (30:Chap. VII)
      1. Legal status of the layman offering first aid treatment. Diagnosis and treatment are the responsibility of the medical profession.
      2. Rudiments of first aid as a part of the equipment of the physically educated person. Modern outdoor life requires a knowledge of first aid. The first aid kit—what it should contain.

VIII. The Health Examination.
   A. The purposes of the examination.
      1. For the student's protection.
      2. For determining needs of individual students to which the service program can contribute.
      3. The purpose and procedure of the re-examination required before readmittance to classes after illness or injury.
      4. The examination as an educative device.
   B. The office of the school physician and its relationship to the conduct of the physical education program.

IX. The Organization of the Service Program and Related Divisions of the Physical Education Department of the Institution.
  A. The service program, including activities, units of instruction, orientation, introductions, and appreciations.
  B. Intramural activities.
  C. Intercollegiate athletics.
    1. Freshman teams.
    2. Varsity teams.
    3. Membership in a conference.
      a. Other schools in the conference.
      b. Eligibility requirements of athletes.
      c. Rules and regulations of the conference.
      d. Conference meetings: why, when, and where held.
      e. Faculty control of athletics.
      f. What other conferences are doing regarding the so-called overemphasis of athletics, subsidization, etc.
    4. Athletic awards.
      a. Freshman numerals, how earned and awarded.
      b. Varsity letters and other awards.
      c. The Block Letter Society.
    5. The athlete as a representative of the student body.
    6. How to come out for a squad.
  D. Teacher training in physical education. A profession.*
    1. The types of positions available. (9:24)
    2. The origin, history, development, and trends of the profession.
    3. Personal qualifications necessary for success.
    4. Training and experience necessary.
    5. Cost of preparation—opportunities to "work one's way."
    6. Salaries to be expected.
    7. Opportunities for advancement.
    8. Working conditions, hours, etc.
    9. Demands upon the vitality of the teacher in this field.
    10. Community relationships of the teacher.
    11. Other related information and materials.

X. The Olympic Games. (1) (15)
  A. The origin, development, and history of the Olympic Games. The Olympic Ideal.

* This unit is, in a sense, a form of vocational guidance.

B. The international committee and how it functions.
C. The organization in America.
D. Activities included in Olympic competition.
E. Meters versus yards.
F. Interesting highlights of the Olympic Games.
G. Amateurs versus professionals.

Summary

The suggested outline presents some material for instruction in the introductions and appreciations course. Teachers of this course would soon develop other materials. The materials indicated have been tried in an actual teaching situation and have been found practical, interesting, and contributive to the needs of students for an all-round introduction to and appreciation of physical education.

In the course in introductions and appreciations, physical education should be discussed in such a manner that significant relationships can be seen in their true proportions. Upon the completion of the course, students will have a knowledge and understanding of objectively determined backgrounds, purposes, and values of physical education. They will be equipped with a sound background upon which to make judgments regarding participation in the school program of physical education and in the community program of recreation. They will, in short, be educated and intelligent in regard to the *why* of participation in physical education pursuits as students, and as adults.

Many pressing problems of athletics and community recreation await an intelligent public opinion. Williams[5] states that the distressing problems of professionalism in athletics can be met partly by educating the alumni of institutions but that this must be done while they are undergraduates. Extended facilities and personnel for physical education will be obtained only when the voting population knows the values inherent in properly conducted physical education pursuits. It is expected that participation in a course in introductions and appreciations of physical education will, in time, bring about these reforms by

[5] Williams, J. F. *Op. cit.*, 1938, p. 295.

raising the intelligence and appreciation of the people of America regarding this significant phase of the curriculum of educational institutions.

SOURCES

1. Menke, Frank G. *The All Sports Record Book*. The All Sports Record Book Co., 235 East 45th Street, New York.

   Gives the origin, history, records, and the highlights of all sports in America. Draws many comparisons between the several sports, their popularity, attendance, etc. Published annually.

2. The American Association of School Administrators. *Youth Education Today*. Sixteenth Yearbook. Washington, D. C., 1938.

   An excellent treatment of the problems of youth today in contemporary American society. Lists the organizations that are concerned with the youth problem and the problems that are being attacked through organized education and related agencies.

3. The American Red Cross. *Life Saving and Water Safety*. P. Blakiston's and Sons Co., Inc., Philadelphia, 1937.

4. The American Red Cross. *First Aid Textbook*. P. Blakiston's and Sons Co., Inc., Philadelphia, 1937.

5. Cozens, F. W. *Achievement Scales in Physical Education Activities for College Men*. Lea and Febiger, Philadelphia, 1936.

   Groups college men into nine normal classifications according to height, weight, and body build. Has achievement scales for a large number of college physical education activities.

6. Cozens, F. W. and Nixon, E. W. *Introductions to Physical Education*. W. B. Saunders Co., Philadelphia, 1934.

7. Dewey, John. *Experience and Education*. The Macmillan Co., 1938.

   The newest work of Dewey regarding the purposes and conduct of education in the light of the philosophy he has made so essential to modern education and its place in American life. Short and understandable.

8. Educational Policies Commission. *The Purposes of Education in American Democracy*. Washington, D. C., 1938.

   Discusses the purposes of education under four main headings. Many of the objectives of health and physical education can be drawn from this source.

9. Elliott, Ruth. *The Organization of Professional Training in Physical Education in State Universities*, p. 44. Bureau of Publications, Teachers College, Columbia University, New York, 1927.

10. Fishbein, Morris. *Shattering Health Superstitions*. The Liveright Publishing Co., New York, 1934.

   Discusses many health superstitions and exposes them in the light of modern medical knowledge. Very interesting and enlightening.

11. Hopkins, L. T. et al. *Integration—Its Meaning and Application*. D. Appleton-Century Co., New York, 1937.

   An excellent discussion of integration. Tells what integration really is,

Shows that modern education must be oriented in the problems of living of each student as an individual.

12. Howard, Glenn W. "The Possibility of Enriching Instruction in the Service Courses." *Proceedings of The College Physical Education Association,* 1937.

13. Hughes, W. L. and Stimson, Pauline E. "Motion Pictures in Health and Physical Education." *Research Quarterly,* Vol. IX, No. 1, March, 1938.
    Outlines the educational significance of motion pictures as supplementary instruction in health and physical education. A comprehensive guide to available films in the United States. Also, the films are classified according to activities.

14. Hughes, W. L. *Administration of Health and Physical Education in Colleges.* A. S. Barnes and Co., New York, 1935.
    Discusses the orientation movement in college physical education. Explains its historical backgrounds, present practices, and its organization and administration in college departments.

15. Kiernan, John. *The Story of the Olympic Games.* Frederick A. Stokes Co., New York, 1936.
    The complete story of the Olympic Games from 776 B.C. to A.D. 1936. Profusely illustrated. Includes the most interesting highlights of the ancient and modern games, the activities performed, the Olympic Ideal and its reinterpretation in modern times.

16. Leonard, F. E. and McKenzie, R. T. *A History of Physical Education.* Lea and Febiger Co., Philadelphia, 1927.
    A complete history of physical education. Gives the background of physical education in America and the sources from which it has been drawn. The various purposes, systems, and organizations of physical education are clearly discussed.

17. Little, L. and Harron, R. *How to Watch Football: The Spectator's Guide.* McGraw-Hill Book Co., New York, 1935.

18. Lloyd, F. S., Deaver, G. D., and Eastwood, F. R. *Safety in Athletics.* W. B. Saunders Co., Philadelphia, 1936.

19. McCormick, Hubert J. "Orientation in Physical Education." *The Journal of Health and Physical Education,* March, 1940.

20. The Phi Delta Kappan. "Teaching As a Man's Job." *Phi Delta Kappan,* Homewood, Ill., 1938.
    A vocational analysis of the teaching profession for men. States the qualifications of teachers, preparation necessary, chances for advancement, salaries, and the obligations and the challenge to a teacher as a member of a profession.

21. Rugg, Harold. *American Life and the School Curriculum.* Ginn and Co., Boston, 1936.
    Shows that the curriculum must be vital and functional and that the problems of daily American life constitute the bases from which the curriculum must be drawn.

22. Schneider, E. C. *Physiology of Muscular Exercise.* W. B. Saunders Co., Philadelphia, 1939.

23. Sharman, Jackson R. *An Introduction to Physical Education.* A. S. Barnes and Co., New York, 1934.
    A textbook for an introduction course in physical education.

24. Sharman, Jackson R. *Modern Principles of Physical Education.* A. S. Barnes and Co., New York, 1939.
25. Williams, J. F. *Exercise and Health.* The National Health Series. The National Health Council, Edr. Funk and Wagnalls Co., New York, 1937.
26. Williams, J. F. *Principles of Physical Education.* W. B. Saunders Co., Philadelphia, 1938.

    Indicates the sources from which the principles of physical education are derived and shows that principles are subject to change as the data change. This reference has long been the "Bible" for all physical educators, regardless of the school level with which they are identified.
27. Williams, J. F. and Brownell, C. L. *The Administration of Health and Physical Education.* W. B. Saunders Company, Philadelphia, 1939.

    The best source of administrative procedures in physical education. Lists the organizations in America that are identified with the various related fields and explains organization and procedures for the administration of all phases of physical education.
28. Williams, J. F. and Hughes, W. L. *Athletics in Education.* W. B. Saunders Co., Philadelphia, 1934.

    Shows the relationship of athletics to the educational curriculum as a whole. Gives the history of athletics and practices to be avoided, and outlines the proper organization for its administration in colleges.
29. Williams, J. F. and Nixon, E. W. *The Athlete in the Making.* W. B. Saunders Co., Philadelphia, 1932.
30. Williams, J. F. and Morrison, W. R. *A Textbook in Physical Education.* W. B. Saunders Co., Philadelphia, 1939.

    A textbook devised for use in elementary courses in physical education in colleges.
31. Williams, J. F., Dambach, J., and Schwendener, N. *Methods in Physical Education.* W. B. Saunders Co., Philadelphia, 1939.

    An excellent discussion of the application of the principles of physical education to teaching method.

CHAPTER VI

The Supplementary Program: Instruction Units

THE physically educated person needs to have an understanding and appreciation of the sports of America. An increasing part of the free time of educated persons is being devoted to physical recreation. It is one of the primary purposes of the physical education service program to prepare students to become proficient while they are in school in several team and individual or dual sports which can be used as recreational sports both in school and out of school. But there are many sports on the American recreational calendar. Students must be encouraged to gain proficiency in those which appear to fit in best with their patterns of needs.[1] Few students have either the time or the ability to master a large number of activities. On the other hand, one of the major purposes of education is to prepare people to become intelligent spectators, as well as creditable performers in a number of sports.[2]

In preparing students for better and more intelligent living in regard to physical education activities, there appear to be two principal needs:

1. The development of skill of performance in several team and several individual or dual sports to the point where pleasure is derived from their pursuit.

2. The development of a knowledge and understanding of the backgrounds, purposes, conduct, and values of each activity that is pursued as well as of the majority of the sports that will be witnessed as a spectator, read about in the sports pages, or discussed with others.

[1] See: Chapter III.
[2] Educational Policies Commission. *The Purposes of Education in American Democracy*, pp. 50, 63. National Education Association, Washington, D. C., 1938.

It is with the second of these needs that this chapter is primarily concerned. How can opportunities be provided in the physical education service program for students to gain a knowledge and understanding of sports in order to be intelligent regarding them as a non-performer? Here again it seems desirable to supplement instruction in connection with each of the activities of the program by means of discussions, readings, and written materials.

In addition to actual physical skills in the performance of a given activity, the following factors seem to fall within the realm of "spectator" needs in connection with an activity:

1. The origin, history, development, trends, and place of the activity in American life, and, consequently, in the curriculum of educational institutions.

2. An understanding of the principal rules of the sport, together with the reasons for their establishment.

3. Possible modifications of rules, equipment, and playing areas so that the game can go on in situations where there are smaller or larger numbers of participants, unofficial playing areas (picnics, socials, etc.), or coeducational participation.

4. The selection, purchase, and care of sport clothing and sport equipment.

5. A knowledge of what "good form" is in the performance of the activity as well as an understanding of the effect of individual differences in ability to achieve good form.

6. The etiquette of the sport for participant and spectator.

7. How schedules are arranged in connection with the sport. (Seeding, handicapping, types of tournaments, i.e., round robin, elimination, match, medal, etc.)

8. How to read and interpret the sport page in regard to the sport. A working knowledge of the terminology of the game.

9. In vigorous bodily-contact sports one should know of common injuries, how to avoid them, and how to treat injuries.

10. Appreciations of the activity, including:
    a. Its place in the curriculum.
    b. Its value as a carry-over recreational sport.
    c. Determination of a "self par" as a standard by which to judge personal success or failure of performance.

A broad interpretation which considers physical education as preparation for life, as *education* rather than mere *physical training,* indicates that materials such as those included in the list point out areas of student needs too important to be left to mere chance. It is too much to hope that a knowledge and understanding of these materials will be acquired concomitantly with physical performance of the activity. It seems advisable to devote some time to discussion, assignments, and examinations in regard to them. The amount of time to be devoted to this phase of instruction will vary with the materials to be included. For an activity class meeting three times a week, it is suggested that one weekly period be devoted to discussions, demonstrations, motion pictures, assignments, and examinations covering both the physical technics and the related learnings.

Outlines of instruction units for two activities—golf and tennis—are presented here. In addition to instruction in the technics and skills, students should submit written reports covering the questions which appear in each unit. Whenever possible, they should be encouraged to outline answers briefly so that the papers can be easily read and marked. Such materials, when read, marked, and returned to students, should be discussed. In this way each unit becomes a valuable teaching device.

GOLF

It is a science—the study of a lifetime, in which you may exhaust yourself but never your subject. It is a contest, a dual or melee, calling for courage, skill, strategy, and self-control. It is a test of temper, a trial of honor, a revealer of character. It affords a chance to play the man and act the gentleman. It means going into God's out-of-doors, getting close to nature, fresh air, exercise, a sweeping away of mental cobwebs, general recreation for the tired tissues. It is a cure for care—an antidote for worry. It includes companionship with friends, social intercourse, opportunity for courtesy, kindliness, and generosity to an opponent. It promotes not only physical health but moral force. DAVID R. FORGAN

Unit One—Orientation

1. Where did golf originate and how did it come to the United States? (2) (4:146)*
2. Name the three grips used in golf. What are the functions of a grip? Which grip seems to be most universally used? (1a) (4:154) (7:1) (5) (6)

* The first number in parentheses refers to the reference in the bibliography on page 95. The second number refers to the page in the specified reference.

3. Explain how one "lines up" and "addresses the ball" with:
   a. The putter.
   b. Irons.
   c. Woods. (1a) (7) (5) (3)
4. Name the lengths of golf clubs? Clubs made to the measure of the individual player are called what? Why should one buy from an "open set" of golf clubs? (10)
5. From what part of the club does the number come? What is the "face"? The "sole"? The "heel"? Can both woods and irons have the same number? (6:5)
6. What is meant by "stance"? Explain by diagram what is meant by a "square stance"? An "open stance"? A "closed stance"? (6:13) (7:5) (4:154)
7. What is the most significant factor in determining par for a hole? What other factors are there? (9:89) (8:302)
8. What national associations promote golf in America? Are there any international associations promoting golf? (2) (9)
9. What is "medal play"? "Match play"? (9) (10) (8:300) (6:67)
10. When may one "tee off" if a party is in the fairway you wish to use? What does the rule state about approaching a green when another party is putting on it? (9:55) (10)
11. Name five terms peculiar to golf. (10) (Appendix)
12. Which phase of golf (woods, irons, putter) is most used?
13. How does the term "away" indicate who shall shoot next in golf? (10) (9:55)
14. Why is golf referred to as a carry-over sport? What factors favor such a carry-over? (10)

Unit Two—Putting

1. Discuss the statement: "Although there are almost as many styles of putting as there are golfers, there are certain principles of form common to all good putters." (10)
2. Explain how to "line up" for a putt. (1a:51) (7:27)
3. Is it possible to "hook," "slice," or "top" a putt? (10)
4. Why is it desirable to have the two hands work together as one when putting? (5) (7)
5. Is putting done primarily with a wrist action or an arm swing? Is any arm movement desirable in putting? (6: Chapters III and IV)
6. How many putts are "par" for a green? (See: Unit One—Question 7)
7. Where should one lay the flag when putting? His golf bag? (10) (Appendix)
8. What is the relationship of a "stymie" to match and medal play? (9)
9. What should one aim at when putting? (10)
10. What is the size of the cup? (9)
11. When may a putt be legally conceded? (9)
12. Do the rules permit the use of a putter except on the greens? (10)

Unit Three—Tee Shots*

1. What is meant by the term "a full swing"? (7:8) (1a)
2. Show by diagram the proper way to line up and address a ball for a tee

* This term includes all shots from the fairway with the wood clubs and also full-swing iron shots. In working out this unit, one should become familiar with

shot. Indicate the line of flight, the position of the ball, and the position of the feet. (1a:41) (7:17) (3)

3. Explain how you determine the distance your body should be from the ball as you assume your stance and address. (1a:41) (7:17)

4. How high should the ball be teed up for the tee shot? May one shoot from any part of the tee he wishes? How do you determine from where you may shoot? (9)

5. How long should one wait for the party ahead before teeing off? Does the answer you give hold true if one of them is looking for a lost ball? If a tee shot goes out of bounds what is the rule? What is the rule covering a lost ball? (9) (10) (Appendix)

6. Why is it so essential for the left arm to be kept straight when executing a stroke? What happens to the club head if one looks up before the down swing is completed? (10)

7. What is meant by a "pivot"? Explain how a pivot enables one to get the club back in the full swing position at the top of the backswing. (7:Chapter 3)

8. During the backswing, at what point should the wrists begin cocking? (7:Chapter 3) (1a)

9. Should the backswing be fast or slow? Why? (10)

10. At the top of the backswing, in what position should be the individual's head?

11. What should be the position of the right elbow during the swing? (7:opposite page 11)

12. During the downswing at what point should the wrists begin to uncock? Explain how the wrist action can be blended in with the arm swing to make up the smooth swing so essential to a successful swing. (6) (1a) (7:Chapter 3)

13. What are the common causes of slicing? Of hooking? Of topping the ball? (7) (1a)

14. In order to be perfectly safe and not bother the shooter where should persons in the foursome stand while one of their party is teeing off? (10) (Appendix)

15. Why is it essential for one to know the distance which can be obtained by a given club with a full swing? Number your clubs and indicate what distance you consistently expect from each. (Men: 4:157) (Women: 6:5)

Unit Four—Approaches†

1. Explain what is meant by full swing, one-quarter, one-half, three-quarters. (6:30–37)

2. Does a modified swing require a shorter grip on the club? If so, why? (10)

3. Why is it necessary to use a modified swing (not a full swing) on some shots? (10)

4. In using a modified swing, how does one determine what distance will be achieved with a given club and a given stroke? For instance, a 6 iron and a one-half swing. (10)

---

the technic involved in the full swing, including stance, address, backswing, downswing, and the follow through. The instruction periods will serve as a laboratory where actual participation of these technics can be learned and checked.

† Approaches requiring a modified swing, i. e., one-quarter, one-half, or three-quarter swing.

5. Does an open stance seem advisable for modified shots? If so, why? (10)
6. What factors determine whether it is best to "pitch and run" or to execute a high shot with considerable backspin when approaching a green? (10) (7:24–26)
7. About how high should one raise the club head during the backswing for a fifteen-yard approach? (6:30)
8. Discuss the statement: "In many respects the short approach, say 15 yards, is similar to putting." List the points of similarity. (10)
9. In short approaches for what should one aim? The green? The cup? (10)
10. What is a "chip shot"? In executing a chip shot can one "follow through" and still get the desired "backspin" on the ball? Explain. What club would you use? Why? (6:26)
11. Is there a pivot and shift of body weight during the execution of short approach? Explain. (7:Chapter VI)

Unit Five—Miscellaneous Shots*

I. SAND TRAPS
1. Why do the rules state one may not ground a club when addressing a ball in a sand trap?
2. There are two principal shots from a sand trap: the "chip" and the "explosion." Under what circumstances would either be advisable?
3. Why is a strong follow through so essential in an explosion shot?
4. Why should one fill up footprints and holes made in a sand trap before leaving it?

II. UPHILL—DOWNHILL—SIDEHILL
1. Should one aim straight ahead, or to the right or left when executing a shot from an uphill lie? Why?
2. Why is it difficult to get a ball to rise when hitting from a downhill lie?
3. If the ball lies on a sidehill below one's feet, why is it advisable to use a long club?
4. If the ball lies above one's feet where should one grip the club? Why?
5. Should distance, or accuracy be the aim when shooting from a difficult lie?

III. ROUGH
1. Discuss the statement: "When playing from the rough it is generally urged that one should try to get back on the fairway even though distance must be sacrificed."

IV. WIND
1. In what way can one take advantage of a "tail wind"?
2. How would a strong "head wind" modify one's game? A "cross wind"?

Unit Six—Appreciations

I. TOURNAMENTS
1. Explain how "pairings" are made in tournament play. (1c:2)
2. How is a ladder tournament conducted? (1c:10)
3. What is a "can you take it" tournament? (1:17) What steps should be

* Thomson, Ben. *How to Play Golf.* Prentice-Hall, New York, 1939. Discusses miscellaneous shots very clearly. Best single reference.

taken before staging such a tournament in order to be sure that participants not in the contest will not be offended?

4. Describe a flag tournament. (1c:20)
5. Explain what is meant by the following terms:
   a. High ball and low ball.
   b. Best ball and aggregate.
   c. Two ball foursome.
   d. Three ball matches. (1c:30–31)

II. HANDICAPPING

1. What is the purpose of handicapping? (8:303)
2. How does handicapping for match play differ from that of medal play? (8:303–312)
3. Is it possible for a sub-par player to have a handicap? (8:310)
4. In the Calkin's Table what is the maximum handicap permitted? (8:309)

III. THE SPORTS PAGE

1. Define "Out" and "In." (8:311)
2. What is meant by first, second, and third flights? (1c:1–2)
3. Which golf association in America and which one in Great Britain sponsor the "Walker Cup" Matches? How often are they held? (2)
4. What are the functions of the P. G. A.? (2)
5. Distinguish between amateur and professional. (9:84) What is an open championship? Amateur championship? A professional championship? (2) (9)
6. What is the "Curtis Cup"? (2)

IV. GOLF AS A LIFE PURSUIT

1. Why is golf spoken of as a "carry-over" sport? (10)
2. About how many golfers are there in the United States? (2)
3. Discuss the statement: "Golf is a challenging pursuit because it is not too difficult for anyone to learn, yet never so easy that the best players lose interest."
4. Is golf sufficiently strenuous to assure participants adequate physiological results for the maintenance of organic vigor from its pursuit? If so, how often should one play? (10)
5. What is the best assurance that one will continue to play golf when an adult? (10)
   a. A near-by course?
   b. Friends who play?
   c. Skill as a player?
   d. An "interest" in the game?
   e. Play for the health?

V. MODIFIED GAMES OF A GOLF NATURE

1. Describe three games based upon golf which can be played indoors, or in a restricted area. (4) (10)

GOLF EXAMINATION

Directions: Some of the following statements are incomplete. Fill in the blanks with the correct answers. Some of the statements are true; others false. Place a "+" directly in front of the number of the true statements and an "O" in front of the false ones. If any part of a statement is false, mark the statement false. Underline the correct answer where choices are indicated.

READ EACH STATEMENT CAREFULLY AND BE SURE YOU UNDERSTAND IT BEFORE MARKING IT.

1. Golf originated in ....
2. The first golf course in the United States was established at ....
   ....
3. The first clubhouse course consisted of ....
4. The first golf balls were made of ....
5. Name two associations which promote golf in the United States:
   (a) ....   (b) ....
6. Which association sponsors the international Walker Cup and Curtis Cup matches?
7. The Curtis Cup matches are for women only.
8. In the United States there are now about: 50,000   250,000   3,000,000 golfers. (Underline the answer you consider most nearly correct.)
9. What is usually referred to as the "nineteenth hole"? ....
10. "The more pitch there is to a club the shorter the length of the shaft" is a rule which holds true for all irons except the putter.
11. The principal reason why a beginner should buy from an open set of golf clubs is that he can replace a broken club with an identical one.
12. The number of the club is derived from the length of the shaft.
13. The hitting surface of the club is called the "face" and is to be distinguished from the "sole" and "heel" of the club.
14. Woods and irons never have the same number because the shafts of the woods are invariably longer than those of the irons.
15. Distance is the only factor to be considered in determining par for a course.
16. The term "three up" refers to medal play.
17. The stymie rule applies only in match play.
18. A player may legally concede a putt if the ball is within .... of the cup.
19. The term "away" indicates the distance from the cup of the player whose turn it is to shoot.
20. A party may tee off as soon as the members of the party ahead have completed their second shots.
21. According to the rules, a party may approach a green only after the party ahead has finished putting and replaced the flag.
22. The flag and golf bags should always be laid off the green.
23. In lining up for a shot, the first thing to determine is the direction desired.

24. As putting is done primarily with a wrist action a follow-through is not desirable.
25. The size of the cup is ....
26. How many putts are par for a green ....?
27. The par for a green, which allows a certain number of putts for a green, is constant even though par for each hole may vary according to its length and difficultness.
28. If one shoots par golf he will have more tee shots than putts; consequently driving may be said to be the most important part of the game.
29. The most common cause of slicing is ....
....
30. The length of a swing (full, half, etc.) depends upon the distance the club head is brought back on the backswing.
31. The most common cause of topping is ....
....
32. The rules state that a player must replace all "pivots" to keep the course in good condition.
33. Many faults of beginning golfers can be kept to a minimum by keeping the head motionless and the eyes on the ball throughout the entire swing.
34. The principal factor in developing a fast downswing is: strength   a fast arm pull   a fast backswing   the uncocking of the wrists. (Underline best answer.)
35. In spite of the mechanics involved in lining up, in addressing the ball, and in the swing, a neuro-muscular hand-eye co-ordination is necessary for each individual on each stroke. Consequently, the importance of keeping the eye on the ball cannot be overestimated.
36. A half-swing shot will usually result in one-half the distance normally acquired by a full swing with the club in question.
37. The target in short approaches should be ....
38. A golfer should not ground the club in sand trap shots because by so doing he can inadvertently move the ball and consequently be penalized a stroke.
39. Failure to fill up footprints and "blast-holes" in a sand trap may penalize golfers that follow more so than the original offender.
40. When a player has a bad lie far from the green a wood club should be used in order to make up the distance; otherwise the hole will undoubtedly be lost to the opponent.
41. A ball hit from a downhill lie rises more readily than one hit from an uphill lie.
42. A challenged player in a ladder tournament must accept the challenge or forfeit his position.
43. In a two-ball foursome, each player may shoot two balls and receive credit for the score achieved with the lowest ball.
44. As par is carefully determined for each course, it is unfair to handicap a consistent par golfer.
45. Third-flight players usually have a greater number of handicap strokes than do first-flight players.
46. The "nineteenth hole" figures when the terms "out" and "in" are used.

47. The terms "amateur" and "professional" refer to the degree of skill of the players involved.

48. Golf is a healthful pursuit, particularly when the player continuously reflects upon the health values inherent in each round that he plays.

49. To some degree, the practice of "pairing" will guarantee that the best players in a tournament will reach the finals.

50. List several reasons why you consider golf an excellent carry-over sport.

   a. ....

   b. ....

   c. ....

GLOSSARY OF TECHNICAL TERMS EMPLOYED IN
THE GAME OF GOLF*

Addressing the ball—Taking a stance and grounding club.

Approach—A stroke played to the putting green.

Away—Ball farthest from hole—to be played first.

Baffy—A wood club of small, rounded head and extreme loft.

Bent—A grass commonly used in the United States on putting greens.

Birdie—One under the par figure for the hole.

Bisque—A handicap of a stipulated number of strokes to be taken at the option of the player or side receiving the handicap.

Bogey—An arbitrary standard, supposedly based upon average good play; usually five to seven strokes per round higher than par.

Brassie—The fairway club of maximum power, head of wood. Derives its name from protective brass plate formerly used to cover its bottom. In current practice, a No. 2 wood.

Bulge—The convexity of the face of a golf club.

Bunker—A depression or pit, the bottom of which is covered with rough grass or sand.

Bye—Any hole or holes that remain to be played after the match is finished.

Caddie—A person who carries the golfer's clubs.

Cleek—A narrow iron-headed club of little loft.

Club—The implement with which the ball is struck.

Course—Grounds upon which the game is played. Strictly speaking, to be distinguished from seaside "links."

Cup—The receptacle into which the ball is played to complete a hole.

Dead—A ball is said to be "dead" when it lies so near the hole that the "putt" is a dead certainty. A ball is also said to fall "dead" when it does not run after alighting.

Dormie—One side is said to be "dormie" when it is as many holes ahead as there remain holes to play.

Draw—A controlled golfing shot to the left for a right-handed player; to the right for a left-handed player.

Driver—A wood club of maximum power and minimum loft. Used for maximum distance off the tee.

* From Jones, Robert T. and Lowe, Harold E. *Group Instruction in Golf.* The American Golf Institute, 19 Beekman St., New York. Quoted with permission of the authors and the publisher.

Eagle—Two under par for a hole.

Face—First, the slope of a bunker or hillock; second, the part of the club head which strikes the ball.

Fairway—Specially prepared, closely cropped area intended for play between tee and green.

Flat—A club is said to be "flat" when the angle between its face and the shaft is more than ordinarily obtuse.

Fore—A warning cry to any person in the way of play.

Foursome—A match in which two play on each side, playing alternate strokes on the same ball.

Four-ball match—A match in which two play on a side each playing his own ball.

Green—First, the whole course or links; second, all ground except hazards within twenty yards of the various holes.

Grip—First, part of the handle covered with leather by which the club is held; second, the manner of placing the hands on the club.

Half-shot—An indefinite term used to describe a stroke played less than "full-out."

Halved—A hole is said to be "halved" when each side has played in the same number of strokes. A "halved" match is a "drawn game"; that is, the sides have finished even.

Hanging—A "hanging" lie occurs when the ball lies on a downward slope.

Hazard—A general term for bunkers, streams, ponds and the like, as more particularly defined by the rules of golf.

Head—The striking end of the club.

Heel—First, the part of the head nearest the shaft; second, to strike the ball with this part of the club.

Hole—First, the 4¼-inch hole lined with metal into which the ball is played; second, the entire space between each teeing ground and the cup.

Honor—The right to play first from the tee.

Hook—An uncontrolled golfing shot to the left for a right-handed player; to the right for a left-handed player.

Hosel—The metal socket of an iron club into which the shaft is fitted.

Iron—A club made of metal with the face more or less laid back for the purpose of playing shots of varying distances.

Lie—First, the angle between the shaft and the sole of the club, either flat or upright, as this angle becomes more or less obtuse; second, the situation of a ball, good or bad.

Like—A player is playing "the like" when he is making on a hole a stroke equal in number to that just played by his opponent.

Links—Grounds upon which golf is played. Strictly speaking, the designation is applied only to seaside terrain.

Loft—First, to elevate the ball; second, angle of pitch of the face of the club.

Mashie—An iron club of intermediate loft. According to current practice, a No. 5.

Match—First, the sides playing against each other; second, the game itself.

Match play—Competition by holes won or lost.

Medal play—Competition by total strokes required for the round or rounds provided to be played.

Nassau—A system of scoring awarding one point for the winning of each "Nine" and an additional point for the match.

Neck—The point at which the shaft joins the head of the club.

Niblick—An iron club of greatest loft designed for play from hazards or for short pitching.

Nose—The point or end of the head of the club.

Odd—A player is playing the "odd" when on a given hole he is making a stroke one more in number than that last played by his opponent.

Par—An arbitrary standard of excellence fixed according to length of hole being played; that is, under 250 yards par 3, from 250 to 450 yards par 4; from 450 up, par 5.

Press—To attempt to hit beyond one's normal power.

Putting—The play on the specially prepared surface surrounding the hole.

Putter—A club specially designed for this department of the game.

Rough—Long grass found on that part of the course not specially prepared for play.

Rub of the green—An interference with a ball in play for which no penalty is incurred but whose consequences must be accepted.

Sclaff—When the club-head strikes the ground behind the ball and follows on with a ricochet.

Set—A full complement of clubs.

Shank—The point at which the hosel of an iron club joins the face; a ball struck by the club at this point is said to be "shanked."

Single—A match in which one player opposes one other player, each playing his own ball.

Slice—A golfing shot to the right for a right-handed player and to the left for a left-handed player.

Sole—The flat bottom of the club-head.

Spoon—A wooden-headed club of greater loft than either driver or brassie. In current practice a No. 3 or No. 4 wood.

Spring—A degree of suppleness of the shaft.

Square—When the game stands evenly balanced, neither side being any holes ahead.

Stance—The location of the player's feet when addressing the ball.

Stroke—Any forward motion of the club-head made with the intent of striking the ball.

Stymie—When an opponent's ball lies in the line of a player's "putt." A stymie may occur only in a singles match at match play.

Tee—First, the pat of sand or peg by which the ball is elevated before striking from the teeing ground; second, the teeing ground itself.

Threesome—A match in which one player playing his own ball opposes two others playing alternate strokes on the same ball.

Toe—Nose of the club.

Top—To hit the ball above its center.

Upright—A club is said to be "upright" when the angle between its face and the shaft is less than ordinarily obtuse.

APPENDIX B. GOLF ETIQUETTE

1. Be silent and motionless while another player makes a shot.
2. The best place to stand is diagonally away from a player as he faces the ball; in front of him and to his right.
3. On the putting green, no one should stand beyond the hole in the line of a player's stroke.
4. Watch your shadow. Keep it off the line of play.
5. Allow the player with the honor (player who has the lowest score on the previous hole) to play before any other player tees his ball.
6. No player should play from the tee until the members of the group ahead are completely out of range; nor play up to a green until the players ahead have holed out and moved away.
7. If you have lost a ball, motion the players behind you to play through and then do not resume your play until they are out of range.
8. If you are playing slowly, motion the party behind you to come through; it is the courtesy of the course.
9. The player farthest from the hole should always be allowed to play first, even though he takes several strokes.
10. Count every stroke, "fans" and all. It is no fun to have a low score unless you really earn it.
11. Do not improve the position of the ball unless the rules are to play "winter golf," which means to tee the ball in the fairway.
12. Report to the office of the course to sign the record and to pay the green fee before starting to play.

Sources

1. The American Golf Institute, 19 Beekman Street, New York. Free materials may be obtained.
    a. Jones, Robert T. and Lowe, Harold E. *Group Instruction in Golf.*
    b. Jones, Robert T. *Rights and Wrongs of Golf.*
    c. Jones, Robert T. *How to Run a Golf Tournament.*
    d. *Motion Pictures on Golf.*
2. *The All Sports Record Book.* Published annually by The All Sports Record Book Co., 235 East 45th Street, New York.
3. Barnes, James M. *Picture Analysis of Golf Strokes.* J. B. Lippincott Co., Philadelphia, 1930.
4. Mitchell, E. D. (Edr.) *Sports for Recreation,* Chapter XI, "Golf." A. S. Barnes and Co., New York, 1936.
5. Morrison, Alex. *A New Way to Better Golf.* Simon & Schuster, New York, 1932.
6. Schleman, Helen B. *Group Golf Instruction.* A. S. Barnes and Co., New York, 1934.
7. Thomson, Ben. *How to Play Golf.* Prentice-Hall, New York, 1939.
8. Williams, J. F. and Morrison, W. R. *A Textbook of Physical Education,* pp. 296–312. W. B. Saunders Co., Philadelphia, 2nd Edition. 1939.
9. *Official Rules of Golf,* 1939. A. G. Spaulding Bros. Co.
10. Class discussions, mimeographed materials, and supplementary units.

TENNIS

Unit One—Orientation

1. Where did tennis originate? What were some of the characteristics of the early game? How did it start in America? (1:22) (8)*
2. What is meant by "Open Face"? "Closed Face"? "Flat Swing"? "Top Spin"? "Flat Drive"? "Volley"? "Slice"? (3:30)
3. What national and international organizations sponsor tennis? (8) (7)
4. Explain how you would select and care for a good racket? (3:27) (2:5) (10:Chapter 1)
5. Why is it so essential for the beginner, as well as the expert, to use official balls that are in good condition? (3:28)
6. Does the code of sportsmanship for tennis players and for participants differ from that of other sports? (2:91)
7. Once a player has adopted a grip is it advisable to adhere strictly to it regardless of the stroke being executed? (5:6) (1:47) (2:11) (10:14)
8. How is a tennis game scored? How many games constitute a set if one player wins them all? How many sets make a match? When should players exchange sides of the net? (7)
9. What should be the height of the net at the center? (7)
10. What differences, if any, is there between the Eastern and Western grips? (3:52) (3:59) (2:Chapter IV)
11. What types of locomotion are the most useful in tennis? Why is it advisable that there be more than one type? (9) (3:Chapter VIII).

Unit Two—The Serve†

1. Which direction should the individual face when starting the serve? Why?
2. At what should the server aim, that is, where should he attempt to have the serve strike in the receiving court? How is this done?
3. Explain how and where the ball should be tossed up when attempting a serve. Should any spin be imparted to the ball as it is tossed up?
4. Should the arm be fully extended, or bent at the elbow, when contact is made with the ball at service?
5. Is the serve a pushing, striking, or throwing motion? Is a follow through desirable after the contact?
6. What is the footfault rule? Is it enforced in tournament tennis? (7)
7. What position should one assume immediately after serving? Should one run to the net immediately after serving?
8. In which direction should the face of the racket point when the ball is struck for the service? Does the grip on the racket have any effect upon this?
9. When serving, at what should one look: The ball? The position of the receiver? The top of the net? The part of the service court for which he is aiming?

* The first number in parentheses refers to the reference in the bibliography on page 101. The second number refers to a page in that reference.
† See any reference in the Bibliography, except 8. Selected references on the serve are (3:78) (2:46) (1:44).

10. Can one be relaxed and still be in instant readiness to serve?
11. In what position should the receiver be? (2:15)

Unit Three—The Forehand

1. What relation does footwork have to a successful forehand stroke? When striking the ball, should the player step forward with either foot? If so, in which direction will the body face at the time of the impact with the ball? (3:Chapter VIII) (2:Chapter VI) (6:35–36)
2. Does one use the same grip for the forehand stroke as for the serve? (2:17) (6:34) (1:56) (3:5)
3. In the forehand stroke when is the racket higher than the point of contact with the ball? Before, or after the contact, or both? (2:Chapter VI) (6:36) (1: opp. p. 56) (1:58)
4. Explain why standing too close to the ball makes a poor forehand stroke. Does this indicate a straight or a bent arm position at the moment the ball is hit with the forehand stroke? How far from the ball should one be at the time the ball is struck? (3:57) (1:58)
5. What is meant by the "follow through?" (6:36) (1:59) (2:21)
6. On what part of the face of the racket should the ball be struck in executing the forehand stroke? (2:23) (3:53)
7. Should the face of the racket be up (open), down (closed), or parallel to the net when executing the forehand stroke? (3:57)
8. At what height should the ball be met at the time of the impact in the forehand stroke? (3:55–56)
9. Should the racket head be held below the wrist when executing the forehand stroke? If so, what type of shot results? (3:57)
10. What position should one immediately assume upon the completion of a forehand drive? (2:15–16)

Unit Four—The Backhand

1. Should one vary the grip for the backhand stroke? (10:41) (10:14–17) (5:25) (3:59) (2:30)
2. Explain what is meant when the statement is made that the backhand stroke is more of a "pull" than a "push." (10:14) (1:69) (5:24)
3. Why is the backhand stroke considered more difficult than the forehand? Is it true that it is more difficult? (3:59) (5:27) (1:68)
4. Assume that a ball is returned to you on the backhand side. How would you get in position to execute a backhand stroke? (1:69) (5:26) (3:61) (10:44–47)
5. Is it true that a backhand stroke is essentially a lefthanded stroke played with the right arm and that the body position should be similar to that of the lefthander executing a forehand stroke? (9)
6. Start in the "ready" position for a backhand stroke and follow the positions of the racket throughout the stroke. (3:61–62) (10:43–47) (2:Chapter VII) (6:39) (1:70)
7. What position should the racket be in at the time of impact with the ball in order to impart a topspin to the ball? (3:61) (2:36) (10:46)

8. Why does one need "plenty of room" when executing a backhand stroke? (10:21) (10:43)

9. Indicate a desirable elbow position for a backhand stroke at the time the ball is struck? (10:22) (2:35)

10. What position should the body be in at the finish of a backhand stroke? (10:46) (2:34)

Unit Five—The Volley

1. What is a volley? (2:60) (3:102)

2. How does one determine when to come up to the net? (6:Chapter VI)

3. What is the correct volleying position (position on the court)? (10:98) (10:104) (3:103–104)

4. Describe five kinds of volleys. (3:102–103)

5. In what way should the grip be changed for the volley? (3:104) (10:101)

6. Give and discuss two principal errors of beginners in volleying. (3:108) (10:Chapter XV)

Unit Six—Lobs, Chops, Slices

1. Give four reasons for using the lob. (3:11)

2. What is a smash? (1:92) What is the purpose of a smash? (10:108)

3. Where should one stand, in relation to the position of the ball, for a smash? (10:112) (2:Chapter XII) (3:Chapter XV)

4. What is a chop? (3:119) For what is it used? (3:119)

5. What is a slice? (3:119) (2:Chapter XIII) For what is it used? (3:119) (2:Chapter XIII)

Unit Seven—Tactics and Strategy

1. What are the two principal styles of playing singles? (4:107)

2. Give four rules that the server should observe in the singles game. (4:110) (2:Chapter XVII)

3. Give four rules that the receiver should observe in the singles game. (4:110)

4. What part of the court should one avoid? (5:89) (2:93)

5. Give two possible positions for players of a doubles team. (5:101) (6:116)

6. Is net play more, or less important, in doubles than in singles play? (5:Chapter VII) (4:122) (6)

7. Give four rules for doubles play. (4:129)

Unit Eight—Appreciations

1. Why is it said that tennis is a carry-over game? What are the characteristics of a carry-over game? (9)

2. Draw up a bracket for an elimination tournament for 8 players. For 10 players. (7) (4:135–139)

3. What is a ladder tournament? (7) (4:142)

4. What is meant by seeding? (7) (4:141)

5. What are the Davis Cup Matches? (8)

6. What are the Wightman Cup Matches? (8)

7. What is an amateur? (7) (5:145)

8. Give six rules of tennis etiquette. (6:Chapter XIX) (3:134) (4:161) Give four rules of etiquette for the spectator. (3:135) (6:154)
9. Give several rules of training for tennis. (6:Chapter XVII)
10. Draw a diagram of an official tennis court (singles and doubles). (7) (5:117)
11. How long should a party continue to play on a court if others are waiting to use it? (9)
12. What are the position and duties of the tennis umpire? May he also keep score? (7) (9)

TENNIS EXAMINATION

Directions: Some of the following statements are incomplete. Fill in the blanks with the correct answers. Some of the statements are true; others false. Place an "x" directly in front of the number of the true statements and an "o" in front of the false ones. If any part of a statement is false, mark the statement false. Underline the correct answer where choices are indicated. READ EACH STATEMENT CAREFULLY AND BE SURE YOU UNDERSTAND IT BEFORE MARKING IT.

1. Tennis originated in ....
2. It was a modification of: Cricket   Table Tennis   Croquet   Handball. (Underline the correct answer)
3. Tennis was originally a game reserved for the aristocracy.
4. The game of tennis came to America by way of Bermuda.
5. Which organization exerts the controlling influence over amateur tennis in America today? ....
6. The award for world's supremacy in tennis for men is called ....
....
7. The award for world's supremacy in tennis for women is called ....
....
8. It is important to use official equipment while learning to play tennis because ....
....
9. The more expensive a racket, the less it is likely to be injured by water.
10. The educated person should know and practice tennis etiquette as a participant and as a spectator.
11. The Eastern grip is undoubtedly inferior to the Western grip.
12. The Western grip is often referred to as the "handshake" grip.
13. Once one adopts a grip it should never be changed for a given stroke.
14. The height of the net at the center should be ....
15. In tournament play, players should exchange sides of the net after each game.
16. Locomotion in tennis is more nearly similar to that of handball than track and field.
17. When serving, the server should face: the net   the right-hand sideline   the left-hand sideline. (Underline correct answer)
18. The ball should be tossed up over the rear shoulder when serving.
19. The footfault rule is seldom called in tournament play.
20. One must step over the baseline and set foot in the court to execute a footfault.
21. One usually should run directly to the net after serving.

22. Serving becomes such a mechanical action that one need not look at the ball when serving.

23. The forehand stroke is similar to a .... motion.

24. The principle of opposition indicates that the right-handed person should step forward with the right foot when executing a forehand stroke.

25. The follow through of a forehand stroke not only assures a better stroke but also places one in a better position for the return shot.

26. It is generally agreed that a forehand stroke should hit the ball at the: top   bottom   middle   of the bounce. (Underline correct answer)

27. When the racket is thought of as an extension of the arm, it may readily be seen that one must not be too close to the ball when executing a drive.

28. The backhand stroke is essentially a left-handed stroke accomplished with the right arm.

29. The backhand stroke is more of a pull than a push.

30. A follow through is not as important after a backhand stroke as it is after a forehand stroke.

31. In executing a volley one should always attempt to contact the ball at the top of the bounce.

32. Volleying is more closely identified with net play than any other phase of the game.

33. The lob, although usually a defensive weapon, can also be used offensively.

34. The smash stroke resembles the serve more than it does the forehand stroke.

35. The smash   chop   slice   lob   is the more powerful stroke. (Underline best answer)

36. The point at the juncture of the service courts is a weak position for a player to be in because it is difficult either to volley or drive from there.

37. Net play is more important in the singles game than in the doubles.

38. Tennis doubles is not truly a team game because only two players are involved.

39. The "seeding" of players ordinarily assures that the best players will meet in the final matches.

40. An amateur is invariably a less skillful player than a professional.

41. Tennis is a strenuous game. One should be fully aware of his own physical-organic status before taking part in tennis as a leisure-time pursuit.

42. The official singles court is .... feet by .... feet.

43. If others are waiting to use a court one should: complete the game   the set   the match   play an hour   before relinquishing the court. (Underline best answer)

44. The tennis umpire should never be allowed to keep score.

45. In a ladder tournament the challenged person must play or forfeit his position on the ladder.

46. Lawn tennis rules do not apply to matches played on hard-surfaced courts.

47. There are cases where it is permissible to reach over the net to spike a ball, but the rules state one must never strike the net.

48. One should come up to the net when the opponent is ....
....
....

49. List four games of a tennis nature:
     1. .... 2. .... 3. .... 4. ....
50. Why is tennis referred to as a sport with a high carry-over value? ....
....
....
....

SOURCES

 1. LaCoste, Jean R. *LaCoste on Tennis.* William Morrow Co., New York, 1928.
 2. Bruce, E. S. and Bruce, B. O. *Tennis Fundamentals and Timing.* Prentice-Hall, New York, 1938.
 3. Driver, H. I. *Tennis for Teachers.* W. B. Saunders Co., Philadelphia, 1938.
 4. Randle, Dorothy D. and Hillas, Marjorie. *Tennis Organized for Group Instruction.* A. S. Barnes and Co., New York, 1932.
 5. Lenglen, Suzanne. *Lawn Tennis.* Dodd, Mead and Co., New York, 1926.
 6. Wills, Helen. *Tennis.* Charles Scribner's Sons, New York, 1928.
 7. *Official Rules of Tennis,* 1939.
 8. *All Sports Record Book,* published annually by The All Sports Record Book Co., Inc., 235 East 45th Street, New York. (Frank G. Menke, Edr.)
 9. Class lectures, discussions, and mimeographed materials.
10. Paret, J. Parmly. *Lawn Tennis—Lessons for Beginners,* Vol. I. Lawn Tennis Library. American Lawn Tennis, Inc., New York, 1926.

CHAPTER VII

The Activity Program

Activities must contribute to needs

THE activities of the service program must be chosen and conducted so that situations which contribute definitely to the needs of students are established. Activities constitute the hub of the physical education program. But they are merely vehicles through which individuals can be better educated for a richer life. The activity program, properly prescribed for each person in relation to his needs and supplemented by situations which will encourage the development of knowledge and understandings, is a truly educational medium. A well-planned program will lead to an appreciation of the place of sport and recreation in life, and consequently will be worthy of inclusion within the curriculum.

Student needs are numerous and varied. It has been pointed out that many needs are general in nature for all students. (See Chapter III.) It is also true that each student will have needs unique to himself as an individual. His past experiences, his present status of achievement, and the area of living for which he is preparing must be considered when aiding him in a choice of activities. This does not mean, however, that each student will constitute a physical education class unto himself. While he may have individual needs, they can be met in group situations. Nor is it possible or desirable to have strictly homogeneous groupings within physical education classes. Life does not present homogeneous groupings, and physical education is one phase of preparation for life. Yet safety indicates that some kind of grouping in certain types of activities is desirable. It also appears psychologically sound to separate the novice and the good performer for competition, as neither too much success nor too much failure is conducive to that pleasure and satisfaction which is so essential to a life carry-over of a sport. Observation by the trained teacher appears a more reliable means of classifying students for activity than the use of time-consuming tests and measurements in isolated skills or muscular strength.

Most of the activities that now form a part of service programs are of benefit to most students. Some will be of more value to a given student than others. Advisers in possession of data regarding the relative worth of the different activities of the program and the patterns of needs of students must see that students are guided to participate in those activities of most worth to them.[1]

Criteria for selecting activities

Ideally, a large number of individual, dual, and team activities should be included in the program in order better to meet the varied needs of students. Actually, the number of activities an institution will be able to offer is determined by the size and number of play areas, by the cost of facilities and equipment, by the number and training of staff members, and by other limiting factors. Therefore, particularly in situations where a wide variety of activities cannot be offered, some criteria for choosing the activities of most worth must be established. Criteria must be in keeping with modern purposes of this area of education. The following points are important:

1. The physical education program must be selected and conducted so that the life needs of students are being met in situations which are for each individual physically wholesome, mentally stimulating and satisfying, and socially sound.[2]
2. The physical education program must be selected and conducted in keeping with proved facts or the best available expert opinion in regard to the place and purposes of physical education as an area of education for life in a democracy. Therefore, each activity must be critically examined in terms of proved principles of physical education.

[1] See: Chapter VIII, pp. 118–123.
[2] Williams, J. F. *Principles of Physical Education,* p. 300. W. B. Saunders Co., Philadelphia, 1938. Quoted with permission of the publisher.

3. Activities must be selected which will result in the greatest benefit for the greatest number of students.

The Committee on Curriculum Research of the College Physical Education Association, in a study of long standing which drew upon the services of many experts in physical education, used five points in evaluating activities:

1. The contribution to the physical and organic growth and development of the child and the improvement of body function and body stability.

   Activities should be vigorous, but not too strenuous. This can only be determined through a thorough knowledge of the physical-organic status of the individual and the degree to which he is trained and conditioned for the activity.

2. The contribution to the social traits and qualities that go to make up the good citizen and the development of sound moral ideals through intensive participation under proper leadership.

   Activities should be sufficiently competitive-cooperative to require the exercise of cooperation, loyalty, courage, perseverance, and other social and moral learnings. Team games are particularly high in potentialities for the development of these qualities.

3. The contribution to the psychological development of the child, including satisfactions resulting from stimulating experiences physically and socially.

   Activities should be interesting, easy to learn, yet challenging enough so that pleasure and satisfaction result as the educative process progresses.

4. The contribution to the development of safety skills that increase the individual's capacity for protection in emergencies, both in handling himself and in assisting others.

   a. Some activities are more hazardous than others, yet have many desirable qualities which make them worth including in the program.

   b. The development of proficiency in fundamental neuromuscular skills is a general contribution to one's ability to handle himself in event of emergencies.

   c. Proper sequence in teaching safety skills in any activity will minimize hazards of injuries.

5. The contribution to the development of recreational skills that have a distinct function as hobbies for leisure-time hours, both during school and in after-school life.

The sports and games which are used daily by Americans at play should be in the program. Individual sports are particularly high in relation to this criterion. This point also involves the learning of the sport or activity beyond the novice stage so pleasure and satisfaction will accompany play. Without this there is little likelihood of carry-over.[3]

Hughes adds another criterion:

"Some activities require costly equipment and large areas, yet serve no more students than others more economical to promote. Some activities are dangerous and hazardous without expert supervision, instruction, and safety facilities."[4]

Another criterion seems advisable:

The major games and sports of America should be included in the program so that students can establish a background of playing knowledge upon which to develop a sound appreciation and intelligent analysis of these activities as spectators. In this connection due regard must be given to community customs and traditions. Usually, however, football (touch), basketball, golf, tennis, swimming, baseball (softball), and possibly swimming and track and field are the major athletic games of America. In some communities one would have to add winter sports: ice hockey, skiing, and others.

These criteria for selecting activities for the service program in physical education are sound. They have been generally accepted by the profession. They are in keeping with the analysis of student needs made throughout this study. In judging the worth of an activity one should consider *all* the criteria. For instance, touch football, while somewhat hazardous and of doubtful value as a carry-over sport, would rate very high when measured against the other criteria because of the values inherent in it. Individual sports are high in carry-over value but do not offer situations which are sufficiently cooperative-competitive to rate very high according to other criteria. Yet a balance of individual and team sports is recommended for the service program.

[3] Committee on Curriculum Research. Headings quoted from *The Physical Education Curriculum*. College Physical Education Association. The University of Southern California Press, Los Angeles, Calif., 1940.

[4] From: *Administration of Health and Physical Education in Colleges*, by W. L. Hughes. Copyright, 1935, by A. S. Barnes and Co., New York, p. 180.

Included in service programs the country over are many activities which meet the criteria established. All have value in that they contribute to student needs. The important thing is to see that each student is guided or assigned to the activities that are of most worth to him in relation to his particular pattern of needs and that the activity is conducted and supplemented so that "whole learning" results. The following activities are suitable for the service program in physical education:

TEAM	CO-EDUCATIONAL[5]
Touch football	Golf
Basketball	Tennis
Softball	Badminton
Volleyball	Swimming
Track and field	Hiking
Speedball	Riding
Soccer	Fishing
	Hunting
INDIVIDUAL OR DUAL	Archery
Swimming	Camping
Golf	Boating
Tennis	Ping Pong
Handball	Shuffleboard
Social dancing	Social dancing
Badminton	Tap dancing
Ping Pong	Bowling
Boxing, wrestling, and jiu jitsu	Skating
Winter sports (regional)	Skiing
Camping and outdoor activities	
Bowling	

Local customs and tradition, student interests, unusual facilities, or the particular training of staff members may warrant the inclusion of other activities. The needs of certain students may also justify other activities or a modification of existing ones.[6]

Interest is increasing in winter sports and outdoor life, with an emphasis on skiing, skating, tobogganing, camping, fishing,

[5] See: Chapter III, p. 48.
[6] See: Stafford, George T. *Sports for the Handicapped*. Prentice-Hall, New York, 1940.

hunting, hiking, riding, and boating. Teacher-training institutions are preparing teachers in these areas.[7] These pursuits comprise a large part of the leisure-time life of the people of America and consequently are well worth inclusion in a physical education service program. There appear to be several possibilities through which such material can be included in the program:

1. Separate, distinct courses in skiing, ice skating, ice hockey, hunting, fishing, boating, camping, and hiking.

2. Combination or survey courses such as:

   A. Winter sports
      Ice hockey
      Skating
      Skiing
      Tobogganing

   B. Outdoor life
      Boating
      Camping
      Fishing
      Hiking
      Hunting

3. Introduction of units within the introductions and appreciations course in which such activities are discussed and illustrated. In this way student interests can be developed. As the interests and appreciations become more definite, the need for separate classes will be apparent.

Regardless of which plan is used in a given situation, instruction should include:[8]

1. The discussion of available areas for participation in outdoor sports, within access of the community.
2. The selection, construction, purchase, and care of equipment.
3. Technics of performance.
4. Safety education in connection with each of the activities.
5. Sources of materials for further study and reference.
6. Standards of conduct for the participant and for the onlooker.

[7] Columbia University Camp Leadership Course. Columbia University, New York. Summer Session Bulletin, Alabama Polytechnic Institute, Auburn, Ala. Summer Session Bulletin, Chico State College, Chico, Calif.
[8] See: Chapter VI.

Survey courses in activities

Recently, physical educators have focused attention on the combination or survey course in physical education. This procedure has been borrowed from other fields of the curriculum. In these courses a number of activities are combined to make up the semester calendar. Usually it consists of team sports, although there is no valid reason why individual and dual activities cannot also be included. The following reasons are offered for such courses:

1. There are many activities in the physical education program with which students should be familiar as participants and as spectators. This procedure makes it possible to present many of these activities in a short time.

2. The procedure consequently brings about maximum benefit to large numbers of students in spite of limitations of staff and facilities.

The following reasons are advanced for making up such a course primarily of team games:

1. Team games afford situations in which large numbers of new students can become better acquainted with each other and have opportunities to develop desirable standards of conduct in highly competitive-cooperative situations. In addition, the students develop an appreciation of the physical skills involved in major sports of America.

2. The development of desirable standards better prepares students to become intelligent, appreciative spectators of sports.

3. Inasmuch as the service program is not considered a "feeder" for the athletic program, an entire term's work in a single sport —in order to gain a high degree of efficiency—is not essential.

4. By giving students an opportunity to experience a number of sports of the team type in the first year of school, they will have more opportunity to choose individual sports for the second year's program. In this way a balance between team and individual sports is gained.

5. The survey course combines well with the supplementary program and is easily organized as a combination classroom-gymnasium or field procedure.

For small institutions, with limited staff and facilities, the survey course is especially valuable. In one instance at least it has been used in a large institution.[9] One objection to the course, however, has been advanced. Students should not be required to repeat courses in which they have had adequate past experiences. Many students, however, benefit from it, because supplementary materials are introduced which enrich their knowledge and appreciation of the activity. Furthermore, as only a short time is devoted to each activity a certain amount of repetition does not seem undesirable, if large numbers of students are benefited by it.

The syllabus

Once selected, a program of activities must never be allowed to become static. Student needs change in degree and emphasis and the purposes of physical education as preparation for modern life must be continually re-examined. New activities will meet criteria and must be included in the program. New teaching methods and materials are constantly being revealed through study, research, and experimentation. Minor revisions of program content and method are continually necessary; major revisions may be necessary. As instructors see the need for revision they should report it in writing, indicate reasons for the contemplated change, and state an opinion as to how the change can best be accomplished. These reports should be filed with the director and discussed at staff meetings. In this way all staff members will have a voice in policy-making through a democratic procedure.

Each instructor is looked upon as a specialist in regard to the activities he teaches. As a specialist, he should be assigned to draw up a syllabus for each of these activities. In some cases two or more instructors who are dealing with the same activities should work together on this project. The syllabi should then be discussed in staff meetings before being drawn up in permanent form. This serves the dual purpose of drawing upon the expert

[9] Davis, E. C. "Study of the Interest of Pennsylvania State College Freshmen in Certain Formal and Natural Activities." *The Research Quarterly*, December, 1933.

opinion of other staff members and of educating them in regard to the purposes, values, and conduct of each of the activities of the program. As each staff member is also an adviser, it is essential that he be able to make a clear judgment regarding the values of each of the activities of the program in order that he can assign students to those areas that are in keeping with their needs. The syllabus should be a rough working guide for instruction and should include the following points:

1. Purposes or objectives of the activity expressed in general rather than specific terms and indicating the several most important contributions it can make to the students.

2. The several principal fundamentals of the activity.

3. The essential rules and regulations of the activity.

4. The major coaching hints, that is, the several most important correct ways of performing the fundamentals which the student must understand before he can begin to work with the activity.

5. The general sequence proposed for the learning of fundamentals.

6. The application of learnings in sequence, according to the semester calendar.

7. The plan of organization for a given period; that is, a rough working estimate of the amount of time that will be spent upon fundamentals, drills, and actual game participation.

8. Indication of the best, most economical, and practical means of arriving at an evaluation of the outcomes of the activity in relation to each student's pattern of needs.

9. A list of relevant references, with annotations.

The syllabus is to serve as a rough guide only. Its purpose is not to determine each specific step of subject matter and class organization in advance. The different individuals, the type of activity, the physical surroundings, and other variables will constantly indicate flexible variations. The syllabus, however, will serve as a guide to action and be something definite from which to work. As the instructor draws it up he crystallizes his thinking in regard to the purposes and values of the activity and the teaching method and sequence through which these purposes and values are best realized. As the syllabi are discussed in staff meetings, all staff members share in this educative process and will develop an appreciation of the program as a whole rather than of a single subject matter phase.[10]

The physical education teacher—an educator

Properly organized and conducted, the physical education service program affords one of the richest fields of opportunity in the entire curriculum of educational institutions. The most important single factor in the establishment of situations which can definitely help to meet the many and varied needs of students in this area of organized education is the well-qualified teacher. A statement of Dean Hawkes is significant here:[11]

"No one else in the entire list of officers, instructors, professors, deans, or presidents begins to have the opportunity to learn and to influence the attitude and fundamentals of living that are current among students as do the athletic coaches and the teachers of health and physical education."

But it is not only with respect to the attitudes of students that the teacher of physical education can contribute. He can aid students to prepare for better living as more intelligent, understanding, appreciative participants and spectators in many of the sports and activities which go to make up such a large part of American life.[12] In order to do so, however, he must be well qualified in regard to the following:

1. A thorough understanding of the backgrounds, purposes, and values of physical education and related fields, such as health and recreation, and the relationships of preparation in these fields to general education and to life itself.

[10] See: Staley, Seward C. and Stafford, George T. *A Sports Curriculum.* The Stipes Publishing Co., Champaign, Ill., for an example of syllabi for a large number of sports included in most physical education programs.

[11] Hawkes, Herbert E. "What Should the Physical Education and Athletic Departments Contribute to the Education of Youth?" *Proceedings of The College Physical Education Association,* p. 13. 1934.

[12] See p. 71.

2. A thorough knowledge of the origin, history, development, and place in the educational program of the several activities in the field of physical education which he is required to teach.

3. An understanding of the application of modern psychological principles to instruction in this field of education.

4. The personality, health, intelligence, appearance, tact, judgment, and other personal qualities considered desirable for the good teacher in any field in the curriculum.

5. A knowledge of the purposes and technics of guidance, including the use of observations, surveys, interviews, rating charts, etc., and the ability to interpret data derived from such sources in terms of student needs.

6. An understanding and appreciation of the needs of students, the relative worth of the different phases of the program to meet these needs, and the ability to encourage students to face the facts and make programs in relation to needs.

7. A knowledge of the purposes and procedures of curriculum-making as these apply to this field of education.

8. The desire and ability to benefit through training-in-service, including participation in professional programs, active membership in professional associations, subscription to the literature of this and related fields, study and schooling on the graduate level.

9. A working knowledge of library technics and library research.

10. Robust health and the ability to stand up under a heavy instructional load which usually consists of some combination of guidance, office routines, coaching of athletic teams, public appearances, and instruction of classroom and laboratory sections in physical education.

It appears that the teacher of physical education cannot develop the skills, knowledge, technics, and understandings that are essential to good teaching in the four-year undergraduate course. In addition to this course, with a major in physical education, several years of experience in teaching and graduate work leading to the Master's degree should constitute the minimum of training and experience for a teacher qualified to participate in the type of physical education program outlined here. It is worthy of note that such well-qualified teachers are available.

The teacher in a program of physical education, such as that outlined in this volume, must continually remember that he is teaching students and not an unchangeable, predetermined, traditional pattern of subject matter. As he teaches these students he, in turn, can also learn with and from them. Participation in the development of a syllabus for the activities he teaches will also be a form of training-in-service and will aid in the unification of the work of the whole department.

CHAPTER VIII

Administrative Problems and Procedures

The requirement

THE practice of requiring participation in college physical education has recently become the subject of much discussion and even considerable controversy. About eighty-five percent of the institutions of college level require participation in a physical education service program for an average of three hours per week for a period of two years.[1] On the other hand, however, in some institutions the requirement in physical education has been abolished but instruction is offered to those students who wish to elect some form of physical education. This group of institutions, it is true, represents a minority at present, but the fact that the requirement has been eliminated in some institutions is significant because it is a movement of recent origin.

It is proposed here that a time requirement should be in effect in college physical education for all students for a period of two years. There appear to be several reasons which justify the requirement:

1. Other subjects of the curriculum are required of students. As physical education, properly organized and conducted, is also of great educational value in the preparation of students for better living, it should be required in order that all students will become better prepared in this area of education.

2. Student needs for physical education learnings are numerous and varied. Because of meager experiences in this area of education in high school and community life, few, if any, students will be found who do not have needs to which the physical education program cannot contribute.

[1] The United States Office of Education. *Physical Education in Institutions of Higher Education.* Pamphlet No. 82. 1939.

3. A physical education program that is well organized and administered is an educational enterprise. In it student needs are determined and situations are set up in order to meet them. Furthermore, individual and group guidance aids students to become aware of their needs in this area. The program aims to help them to become more intelligent and self-directive in regard to physical education pursuits. In order to attain this end, a requirement must be in effect. Upon entrance to college students are not always fully aware of needs. The requirement will insure that needs of students which physical education can help to meet are not being overlooked in the broad education of the whole man.

If, at the end of two years' participation in the service program, the advisory and guidance procedure does not function to the point where students will voluntarily continue with physical education pursuits in regular classes, intramurals, intercollegiate athletics, or community recreation activities, there is little reason for continuing the requirement. This opinion is substantiated by Mitchell.[2] Usually, if the service program has functioned properly and the students have a balance of skills, knowledge, understandings, and appreciations of physical education as a whole as well as of several carry-over sports, they will continue to take part in physical education pursuits after the requirement has been lifted at the end of the sophomore year.

If a requirement is not in effect, many students who are not fully aware of the values of physical education as an area of education which can prepare them for better living will fail to participate. Recent experiences in those institutions where the requirement in physical education had been eliminated show that more than fifty percent of the students failed to elect any form of physical education.[3] Yet student surveys indicate that over ninety-five percent of the students questioned agreed that physical education was of value to them.[4]

If physical education is organized and conducted so that it is

2 Mitchell, Elmer D. "Intramural Relationships," p. 187. *Proceedings of the Society of Directors of Physical Education in Colleges*, 1931.

3 Rider, George L. "Why Have a Physical Education Requirement?" *Proceedings of the College Physical Education Association*, 1934.

4 *Ibid.*

educationally sound, definitely contributive in meeting the needs of all the students, then a requirement is justifiable as long as institutional policy permits requirements in any subject field.

Upper-division students should be allowed to elect physical education for credit if they so desire. They should be encouraged to take advantage of the opportunities offered by the intramural, athletic, and recreational divisions of the physical education program. If problems arise in connection with this voluntary participation, they should be encouraged to consult members of the physical education staff for further advice and guidance.

A number of standards have been proposed regarding the length of the physical education period.[5] Institutional practices establish the standards in most instances. A sixty-minute period is recommended here. Of this, fifteen to twenty minutes is sufficient for the shower and dressing. When activities are conducted close to the shower and dressing rooms, fifteen minutes is sufficient if these facilities are not overcrowded.

For the type of physical education instruction herein recommended, in which instruction in physical skills and technics is supplemented by lectures, discussions, illustrations, readings, assignments, and examinations, it is advisable that physical education classes meet three times weekly with one period a week devoted to the classroom.[6] In the event that use of local community recreation facilities, such as a golf course, riding academy, etc., is counted as a part of the weekly attendance, due adjustment must be made in the college roll books. In addition to requirements for the activity sections of the program, attendance at both the course in introductions and appreciations and the orientation sections should be obligatory on all new students.[7]

Substitution for the requirement

It appears to be a common practice to excuse students from participation in the physical education service program because

[5] See: Williams, J. F. and Brownell, C. L. *The Administration of Health and Physical Education.* W. B. Saunders Co., Philadelphia, 1939.
Also: Hughes, W. L. *The Administration of Health and Physical Education in Colleges,* Chapter VI. A. S. Barnes and Co., New York, 1935.
[6] See: Chapter VI.
[7] See: Chapters IV and V.

of participation in intramural activities, intercollegiate athletics, and military training. In such cases there is a gross misunderstanding of the purposes of physical education in preparing students for life. The intramural program is primarily recreational and provides opportunities to continue with the activities learned in the service program.[8] This participation should be upon a voluntary basis and no credit should accompany it. The intercollegiate athletic program reaches a relatively small number of students. However, athletics demand that a high degree of instruction accompany them. In addition to technics and skills of the particular event or sport, "skull" sessions are held. In these cases being on a freshman or varsity squad should be considered as participation in one of the regular activities of the service program even though the activity is administered by the intercollegiate athletic division of the physical education department. Credit, however, for such participation should be limited to one term. If the student wishes to continue with the sport in other terms it should be considered an elective participation, and no credit should be given for it. There are many activities in the physical education program. In order to become physically educated, one should be a fair performer and have a knowledge and appreciation of several individual activities which he can continue to use upon leaving college. Three years of being on a football squad is not adequate preparation for life in the field of physical recreation.[9]

Similarly, the purposes of military training and physical education are not identical. Neither should ever be substituted for the other.[10]

Close cooperation between divisions within the department of physical education and athletics is essential. In making out programs for men on athletic squads this dual participation must be

[8] Nordly, Carl. *The Administration of Intramural Athletics for Men in Colleges and Universities*, p. 204. Bureau of Publications, Teachers College, Columbia University, New York, 1937.

[9] See: Williams, J. F. and Brownell, C. L. *Op. cit.*, Chapter IX.

[10] See: Williams, J. F. *Principles of Physical Education*, p. 196. W. B. Saunders Co., Philadelphia, 1938.

Also: Clark, H. H. "Administrative Problems in Required Physical Education for Men's Universities." *The Research Quarterly*, May, 1932.

taken into account. Swimming and tennis should be scheduled during the off season for track men. Boxing and football during the same term for the same man are not advisable because of the possibility of hand injuries. Simply because a man is fortunate enough to become an athlete does not lessen his need for a knowledge and reasonable degree of skill in other activities that have a high carry-over value. By exercising good judgment in program making there should be no conflict between participation in athletics and the activities of the service program. Strenuous activities should not immediately precede the hour of athletic workouts. Athletes may be excused from participation in activities of the service program on the day of contests, but attendance at the service classes that day should be required. Too, these players should be required to make up the work missed because of out-of-town trips, as they are required to do in other phases of the curriculum. This might also well hold true in the case of intramural activities.

Repeating courses for credit

It has been stated that there are many activities in the service program in which it is desirable that students gain a reasonable degree of efficiency and acquire a knowledge and appreciation that will continue to function in life. For this reason students should not be allowed to repeat any activity of the service program for credit, any more than any athletic sport as a member of a team. In some cases exceptions may be advisable to make certain that a reasonable degree of skill is acquired. But these cases should be exceptions to the rule and should be permitted only on the request of the student's adviser.

Assigning students to classes

It has been indicated that each student should be aided by an adviser in making a physical education program.[11] It is assumed that students entering college are not well enough informed to make wise choices in regard to those physical education pursuits of most worth to them. They have not had sufficient experiences

[11] See: Chapter II, pp. 17f.

upon which to base a choice. Often they do not know enough about the backgrounds, purposes, and values of physical education, and are not adequately aware of their own needs to which physical education can contribute. Rider[12] points out that the entrance age has been constantly lowered. Students are not sufficiently mature, therefore, to plan their programs intelligently. The high school experiences of students in physical education are of a varied nature, and are likely to be of doubtful quality and quantity.[13] Mere expediency, the influence of friends, or fleeting interests are likely to be the factors which decide choices of physical education pursuits unless competent guidance is afforded.

The normal or "A" group

As stated before, at the time of the health examination all new students are assigned to a physical education adviser.[14] The name of the adviser is written on the classification card.[15] All normal or "A" students are assigned to staff members exclusive of the instructor in charge of corrective physical education. In this manner each staff member will have approximately the same number of normal advisees.

Restricted and corrective or "B" and "C" groups

The restricted and corrective cases ("B" and "C" groups) are assigned to the instructor who directs this part of the program. The school physician must work closely with this staff member and his approval must accompany all activity assignments for these students.

Corrective physical education must never be undertaken without a full understanding of the case and the approval of the school physician. A staff member may supervise the corrective program, it is true, but diagnosis of the defective condition and prescription of treatment thereof are the duties of the physician.

---

12 Rider, George L. *Op. cit.*, p. 130.

13 See: Staley, S. C. "The Four Year Curriculum in Physical (Sports) Education." *The Research Quarterly*, March, 1931.

Also: Wood, T. D. and Cassidy, R. *The New Physical Education*, pp. 182–183. The Macmillan Co., New York, 1931.

14 See: Chapter II, pp. 11–16.

15 See: Chapter II, p. 14.

Ideally, the school physician should also be trained as a physical educator capable of taking over the program of activities for students who are found to have remediable defects.

The "B" division presents a problem because two classifications within it are found. Some students are permanently restricted, while others are convalescing from injury or illness. As soon as a student within this latter group is "normal" again, he can once more be assigned to the activities of the program for normal students. He must, however, be re-examined by the school physician and the change of classification must be approved by him. Therefore, such students are examined upon their return to school after absence due to injury or illness, assigned to the temporary restricted group, re-examined at a later date, and, when fully recovered, reassigned to the normal classification. After each examination a physical education readmit card (Table VII) should be sent directly from the school physician's office to the physical education staff members with whom the student is to take work.

TABLE VII

PHYSICAL EDUCATION READMIT CARD

To Instructor ....

.... has been examined upon his return to school. His condition indicates that he should be assigned to classification:

A   B (Permanent)   B (Temporary)   C

He must be re-examined before any change in classification is made. The re-examination should take place on or about ....

Signed .... M.D.

(School Physician)

Program planning

No new student should plan his program before meeting with his assigned adviser. Because of difficulties that are often encountered in program planning for other subjects, it is essential that advisers be available during the early days of registration. Ideally, advisory sections in physical education should be set in advance of general registration. There are at least two ways in which this can be done:

1. Require all new students to register in advance of old students. Conduct the health examinations, orientation meetings,[16] and physical education advisory sections during this time.

2. Establish an institutional policy which requires all new students to meet a physical education adviser and to make out the physical education program in advance of other courses.

The second plan appears to assume that physical education is more important than other required subjects of the curriculum. In some instances, however, when the general administration is sympathetic toward the attempt being made to meet student needs in the physical education program, this early registration can be effected. The first plan appears to be the better one. New students in most institutions are required to take aptitude tests, intelligence tests, qualifying examinations in certain subject matter fields, and similar measures. Guidance is becoming increasingly more evident in schools and colleges. In order to bring about better guidance, it is reasonable to require new students to take up residence several days in advance of old students. During this period, in addition to the examinations and measurements just indicated, they should take the health examination, attend the general orientation meetings for physical education, and meet with assigned physical education advisers for guidance in program planning in relation to needs.

If student enrollment is large, and the number of staff members limited, the number of students assigned to each adviser in turn will be large. In such cases sections can be organized, or much general instruction in program planning can be given in large groups. Then these groups can be subdivided into smaller units, if the adviser feels this would be practicable. Much worth-while guidance can be accomplished in advisory sections whether they are large, small, or individual.

It is in the advisory sections that the cumulative record card is introduced.[17] Students fill out this card step by step, with the aid

16 See: Chapter IV.
17 See: Chapter II, p. 18.

and supervision of the adviser. Every effort should be made to assist them to plan programs in relation to their needs. Past experiences, life plans, interests, community recreation pursuits, and other measures are recorded and taken into consideration in program planning. When students have completed filling in the data on the card, they should indicate their first preferences with respect to the activities in which they wish to participate. The adviser should then collect the cards, record data from other sources (dean's and guidance department), examine each card carefully, and indicate thereon the activities which appear most desirable for the student. He should arrange a posting of assignments (allowing students to satisfy interests if this seems advisable) and should personally interview those students whose records indicate a need for individual guidance. The adviser should then meet the advisory sections again to explain the meaning of posting of assignments to certain activities, and to give each student an assignment card to the chosen activity. To facilitate program making, an assignment to activities card is shown in

TABLE VIII

ADVISER'S ASSIGNMENT TO ACTIVITIES CARD

First Semester	Second Semester
1.	1.
2.	2.
3.	3.
4.	4.
5.	5.

Note: Your physical education adviser recommends that you take the first activity in the above list for each of the two semesters of your first year in college. If your program positively will not permit this, you should take the second activity appearing on the list and so on down. Present this card to your general adviser who is helping you to plan your whole program.

STUDENT .... ADVISER ....

Table VIII. Several alternative activities should be listed for activities that offer a limited number of sections.

Advisers should be available to students throughout the semester. As the various activities of the program are put in operation, further needs will be determined through observation, interviews, the student's ability in the skills and technics of activities, and the degree to which he develops desirable standards of conduct.[18] Frequently other instructors besides a student's adviser will discover needs of that student. They may offer advice and guidance or send a notation of the needs to the adviser. In this manner each student will be afforded helpful guidance as he moves through the various phases of the service program.

Mid-semester changes of program

It should be administratively possible to transfer a student from one activity of the service program to another at any time during the semester if his pattern of needs indicates that such a change is desirable. After all, the only purpose of administration is to set up situations through which the student needs can be met. If it is found that a student has been assigned to an activity with which he is already familiar and in which he is skilled, a change should be made and he should be assigned to a different activity in which he needs knowledge and skills.

Students who have been through the advisory program for a year, have attended orientation sections, have participated in the class in introductions and appreciations, and have participated in some of the activities of the program should be able to make intelligent choices with respect to the second year's program in physical education. They will have in their possession a background of materials regarding the place and purposes of the whole field of physical education in relation to their own unique needs and life purposes. They will have some knowledge of which types of activities appear to best meet their needs, and, consequently, will be better qualified to be self-directive. Even in the case of second-year students, the cumulative record card should be consulted during program-making. The pattern of activities should be rechecked and the student's choices for the second year duly recorded. When it appears advisable, advisers should be available for personal interviews with second-year students.

18 See Chapter II, "Technics for Determining Student Needs."

Credit

Physical education activity classes which meet three times a week, primarily for skill instructional purposes supplemented by lectures, discussions, assignments, and examinations, have an educational value worthy of more than the one-half unit traditionally allotted to them. If two periods of the three a week are devoted to instruction-participation, an allotment of one unit should be granted. The remaining one period of the week which is assigned to the course in introductions and appreciations of physical education should also have one-unit credit. This latter course is conducted along the same lines as any other course and in view of its educational value should be granted credit.

College curricula are undergoing constant reorganization. Inasmuch as physical education is an integral part of the educational curriculum, it should be given the credit due it. College authorities will need to be made aware of the inherent educational worth of the physical education program before they will consider granting credit to this area on the same basis as any other subject of the curriculum.

Attendance

Institutional requirements regarding attendance should apply to physical education the same as to any field of the curriculum. Students able to attend school can learn something through observation of physical education sections, even if it does not appear advisable for them to take an active part in the activity. In the case of convalescents a modified program is essential.[19] But such students need not be deprived of educational opportunities in physical education any more than they are in any other field of education within the institution. The program can be adapted to their needs.[20] Make-up work for absences should be required in physical education. Excuses for absences should be handled through the regular institutional channels.

[19] See p. 120.
[20] Stafford, George T. *Sports for the Handicapped*. Prentice-Hall, New York, 1939.

Marking

In the program outlined in this volume marking in physical education becomes objective. It is based upon:

1. The student's ability to show improvement in the performance of physical skills and game technics.[21]

2. The development of a knowledge and understanding of the backgrounds, purposes, values, skills, rules, technics, etiquette, etc., of the activity. This knowledge is determined through the use of objective tests as well as through observation of the student's behavior in the activity situations of the program.

3. The degree to which the student participates and contributes to the class discussions.

4. Notebooks or weekly assignments in the activity units.

5. Attendance (upon the institutional basis).

6. Attitude ratings.

It has recently been suggested that grading in physical education should be changed from the traditional letter or number marking system to a brief statement of the student's achievement and a suggestion as to how he can better meet his needs.[22] The cumulative record card affords a place for the adviser's remarks. If the letter or numeral mark is required by the institution, it should be supplemented by a brief statement—if this appears desirable for the individual student in question. The instructor of a given activity should discuss the value of marks with the students in class, pointing out the type of work expected and indicating how the progress of each student is noted during the semester. It is unfair to students to allow them to assume that they are doing fair work and then to give them a poor mark at the end of the term. They should be aware of their status from time to time during the semester. A sample physical education report card is shown in Table IX.

[21] If standardized tests are not used for this purpose, observation charts, such as those illustrated in Chapter II, p. 24, can be used.

[22] Hughes, W. L. "Enriching the Required Service Program in Physical Education." *The Journal of Health and Physical Education*, April, 1939, p. 205.

Also: Cassidy, Rosalind. *New Directions in Physical Education for the Adolescent Girl*, p. 137. A. S. Barnes and Co., New York, 1938.

TABLE IX

PHYSICAL EDUCATION REPORT CARD

STUDENT'S NAME	TERM ....
ACTIVITY	
Section	
Hours	
Days...................	

Improvement in Physical Technic (See Table IV, p. 24) (Determined by Observation and Ratings)	
Average of marks for each unit (See Chapter VI)	
Attendance—Including Score Card for Weekly Play (See p. 124)	
Average of Scores of Attitude Ratings (See Table V, p. 26)	
Average of Marks in Periodical Knowledge Tests (See Chapter VI, pp. 90ff. and 99ff.)	
Mark in Final Examination (See Chapter VI, pp. 90ff. and 99ff.)	
FINAL MARK	
REMARKS	

Library Facilities

The type of physical education instruction outlined in this volume requires adequate library materials for student and teacher alike. In addition to the textbook materials used in the professional field, such periodicals as the *Journal of Health and*

Physical Education, Athletic Journal, Scholastic Coach, and the sports pages of local and regional newspapers should be available to the students in the service program. As these sources will be used by large numbers of students in assigned work, they should be kept on reserve and not permitted to be circulated.

CHAPTER IX

Conclusion

IT HAS been indicated in this volume that the general service program in physical education is in need of enrichment and redirection if it is to assume its rightful place in the curriculum of educational institutions. The service program, properly organized and conducted, provides situations which are truly educative and richly contributive to the needs of students in their preparation for living in this area of life.

It is in the service program that *all* students can take advantage of instruction to develop skills, knowledge, and understandings upon which to base appreciations of forms of physical recreation desirable as life pursuits. The intramural and recreational programs afford opportunities to put these learnings into practice both in school and out of school. This marks the distinction between the service program and the intramural and recreational programs—the former being composed of definitely organized instruction and the latter being primarily of a voluntary recreational nature. It has been pointed out that the intercollegiate athletic program affords opportunities for worth-while educational experiences for *some* students. But this phase of the program is not to be considered as one which offers an adequate preparation for better living in regard to physical education practices. For this reason it must be considered a supplement to the service program, and not a substitute for it.

The proposals of student needs and the establishment of administrative procedures through which these can be met are not entirely new. In this volume, however, an attempt has been made to organize the material in such form and sequence that it will be of value to those who are willing to accept the challenge of enriching the physical education service program so that it will be educational and not merely recreative.

Some would call the type of procedure indicated herein an "individualized program." If one is thinking of a program in which the needs of each student are considered, as the program for that student is planned by the student and the adviser, this would be correct. Students with similar needs will be found in sufficient numbers so that the customary sectioning will still constitute a procedure of college physical education. Even if it were possible, strict homogeneous grouping in physical education would not be desirable. The following opinion expressed by a committee on physical education of the Progressive Education Association illustrates this point:

"If homogeneous grouping were possible, it would have very little to do with a better program in physical education. Better programs call for democratic practice throughout the entire school. This implies granting boys and girls opportunities for significant action in relation to their needs, attitudes, and emergent purposes. These must be experienced by each student in the company of and with the cooperation of, or opposition of, other students. . . . If testing procedures for student classification are to be of value the entire testing procedures now carried on by physical education teachers are of doubtful value. The time so spent could be put to better use through teaching and leadership activities which are more adapted to student needs and purposes."[1]

This does not mean that ability grouping is not advisable. It has been pointed out previously that in bodily contact sports, ability grouping is a form of safety education. In all sports, ability grouping for purposes of competition will provide that reasonable degree of success and failure so effective as a challenge to a continually higher level of performance and a life interest in some form of physical recreation.

The important thing, from the modern educational point of view, is to know that each student is becoming increasingly aware of his own individual status, of the purposes of physical education and physical recreation, and of the significance of the several

[1] The Progressive Education Association, *Physical Education in the Secondary School.* New York, 1938. Quoted by permission of the publisher.

activities of the program to him as an individual with a unique pattern of needs. It is only then that self-direction becomes possible. Only as the student becomes increasingly capable of making intelligent decisions, in the light of true facts, should he be allowed to exercise independence in program making. It is in this way that the desirable carry-over into out-of-school life of the worth-while things learned in college physical education will come about. For this reason, it has been recommended that the requirement, with elective privileges, be continued, but that the program be made so attractive, interesting, and educationally worth while that many students will continue to take advantage of it, both for and without credit, in their upper-class years in college.

Tests and examinations have an important place in such a program. It is through the judicious use of these devices that the self-status of the individual can be determined. The caution is added, however, that the qualities most easily tested and measured are often not the most significant outcomes of physical education.

The well-qualified teacher is an important factor in the whole educational scheme. He should understand the basic principles upon which this area of education is built, and should possess a vast store of human understanding. He should desire to aid students to prepare for life, and should command their respect and cooperation in the guidance and advisory program. For these reasons, the teacher who is familiar with the problems of young people, and who is aware of the outcomes to be derived through physical education pursuits, plays an important part in observing student behavior in the whole situation. He is keenly sensitive to student needs.

The challenge of this modern approach to the physical education profession is a real and stimulating one. It is a challenge to organize and operate physical education pursuits upon the basis of objectives which have been determined from a study of each individual. The "why" of physical education is considered here to be as important as the "how"—if not more so.

It is hoped that the discussions, recommendations, and plans

of organization outlined in this volume will be of value as guides
in the redirection of the college physical education service program. Education in all its phases is undergoing a close and critical appraisal today. Physical education, as a part of the curriculum which can contribute definitely to the needs of *all* students,
has a larger, richer part to play than ever before.

Bibliography

ALLPORT, G. W. *Personality—A Psychological Interpretation.* Henry Holt and Co., New York, 1937.

AMERICAN ASSOCIATION OF SCHOOL ADMINISTRATORS. "Youth Education Today." *Sixteenth Yearbook,* National Education Association, Washington, D. C., 1938.

BLANCHARD, B. E. "A Behavior Frequency Rating Scale for the Measurement of Character and Personality in Physical Education Classroom Situations." *The Research Quarterly,* March, 1932.

BOVARD, J. F. AND COZENS, F. W. *Tests and Measurements in Physical Education.* W. B. Saunders Co., Philadelphia, 1938.

CANNON, W. B. *The Wisdom of the Body.* W. W. Norton and Co., New York, 1932.

CASSIDY, ROSALIND. *New Directions in Physical Education for the Adolescent Girl.* A. S. Barnes and Co., New York, 1938.

CASWELL, H. L. and Campbell, D. S. *Curriculum Development.* American Book Co., New York, 1935.

CHILDS, J. L. *Education and the Philosophy of Experimentalism.* The Century Co., New York, 1931.

CLARK, H. H. "Administrative Problems in Required Physical Education for Men's Universities." *The Research Quarterly,* May, 1932.

COMMITTEE ON CURRICULUM RESEARCH. *The Physical Education Curriculum.* College Physical Education Association. University of Southern California Press, Los Angeles, Calif., 1940.

COZENS, F. W. *Achievement Scales in Physical Education for College Men.* Lea and Febiger, Philadelphia, 1936.

DAVIS, E. C. "A Study of the Interests of Pennsylvania State College Freshmen in Certain Formal and Natural Physical Activities." *The Research Quarterly,* December, 1933.

DEWEY, JOHN. *Experience and Education.* The Macmillan Co., New York, 1938.

DUNBAR, H. F. *Emotions and Bodily Changes.* Columbia University Press, New York, 1938.

EASTWOOD, FLOYD R. "Causes of College Sport Accidents." *The Research Quarterly,* October, 1934.

EDUCATIONAL POLICIES COMMISSION. *The Purposes of Education in American Democracy.* National Education Association, Washington, D. C., 1938.

GLASSOW, R. B. AND BROER, M. A. *Measuring Achievement in Physical Education.* W. B. Saunders Co., Philadelphia, 1938.

GOLDBERG, SAM. "Organic Development Explained for High School Track Teams." *The Athletic Journal,* May, 1937.

HALDANE, J. S. *Organism and Environment.* Yale University Press, 1930.

HALL, BOWMAN. "Training for Middle Distance Runners." *The Scholastic Coach,* March, 1938.

HAWKES, HERBERT. "What Should the Physical Education and Athletic Departments Contribute to the Education of Youth?" *Proceedings of the College Physical Education Association*, 1934.

HAYNES, WILMA. "After College, What?" *The Research Quarterly*, March, 1931.

HERMANCE, GILBERT. "The Nature and Scope of Orientation Courses in Physical Education." *Proceedings of The College Physical Education Association*, 1937.

HETHERINGTON, CLARK. *The School Program in Physical Education.* The World Book Co., Yonkers-on-Hudson, 1922.

HOWARD, GLENN W. "The Possibility of Enriching Instruction in the Service Courses." *Proceedings of the College Physical Education Association*, 1937.

HUGHES, W. L. *Administration of Health and Physical Education in College.* A. S. Barnes and Co., New York, 1935.

HUGHES, W. L. "Enriching the Required Service Program." *The Journal of Health and Physical Education*, April, 1939.

JENNINGS, H. S. *The Biological Basis of Human Nature.* W. W. Norton and Co., New York, 1930.

JONES, ARTHUR J. *Principles of Guidance.* McGraw-Hill Book Co., New York, 1934.

LAPORTE, W. R. (Editor). *The Physical Education Curriculum.* The University of Southern California Press, Los Angeles, 1940.

LINK, HENRY C. "Four Personality Traits of Adolescents." *The Journal of Applied Psychology*, Vol. XX, 1936.

LINK, HENRY C. *The Re-discovery of Man.* The Macmillan Co., New York, 1938.

LITTLE, LOU AND HARRON, R. *How to Watch Football—The Spectator's Guide.* McGraw-Hill Book Co., New York, 1935.

McCLOY, C. H. "Character Building through Physical Education." *The Research Quarterly*, October, 1930.

McCORMICK, HUBERT J. "Orientation in Physical Education." *The Journal of Health and Physical Education*, March, 1940.

MENCKE, FRANK (Editor). *The All Sports Record Book.* Published annually by The All Sports Record Book Co., Inc., 235 East 45th Street, New York.

MITCHELL, E. D. (Editor). *Sports for Recreation.* A. S. Barnes and Co., New York, 1936.

MITCHELL, E. D. "Intramural Relationships." *Proceedings of The Society of Directors of Physical Education in College*, 1931.

MITCHELL, ED. AND MASON, B. S. *The Theory of Play.* A. S. Barnes and Co., New York, 1937.

NORDLY, CARL. *The Administration of Intramural Athletics for Men in Colleges and Universities.* Bureau of Publications, Teachers College, Columbia University, New York, 1937.

PUTNAM, HAROLD (Editor). *The Dartmouth Book of Winter Sports.* A. S. Barnes and Co., New York, 1939.

RIDER, GEORGE L. "Why Have a Physical Education Requirement?" *Proceedings of The College Physical Education Association*, 1934.

RUGG, HAROLD. *Culture and Education in America.* Harcourt, Brace and Co., New York, 1931.

SCOTT, H. A. "Physical Education and Exercises for Business Men." *The Nation's Health*, Vol. IX, No. 6, June, 1927.

SEFTON, ALICE A. "A Guide to the Literature of Physical Education including Certain Aspects of Health Education and Recreation." *The Research Quarterly*, Vol. VI, No. 4. December, 1934.

SHARMAN, JACKSON. *Modern Principles of Physical Education*. A. S. Barnes and Co., New York, 1937.

STAFFORD, GEORGE T. *Sports for the Handicapped*. Prentice-Hall, New York, 1940.

STALEY, SEWARD C. "The Four-Year Curriculum in Physical (Sports) Education." *The Research Quarterly*, March, 1931.

STALEY, SEWARD C. AND STAFFORD, GEORGE T. *A Sports Curriculum*. The Stipes Publishing Co., Champaign, Ill., 1938.

STRANG, RUTH. *Counseling Technics in College and Secondary School*. Harper and Brothers, New York, 1937.

UNITED STATES OFFICE OF EDUCATION. *Physical Education in Institutions of Higher Education*. Pamphlet No. 82, Washington, D. C., 1938.

UNIVERSITY OF CHICAGO LABORATORY SCHOOLS. *Physical Education and the Health of School Children*. Publication No. 5, May, 1936.

VOLTMER, E. F. AND ESSLINGER, A. A. *The Organization and Administration of Physical Education*. The F. S. Crofts and Co., New York, 1938.

WATSON, GOODWIN, COTTRELL, D. P., AND LLOYD-JONES, E. M. *Redirecting Teacher Education*. Bureau of Publications, Teachers College, Columbia University, 1938.

WILLIAMS, J. F. *Principles of Physical Education*. W. B. Saunders Co., Philadelphia, 2nd edition, 1932; 3rd edition, 1938.

WILLIAMS, J. F. AND BROWNELL, C. L. *The Administration of Health and Physical Education*. W. B. Saunders Co., Philadelphia, 1938.

WILLIAMS, J. F. AND HUGHES, W. L. *Athletics in Education*. W. B. Saunders Co., Philadelphia, 1936.

WILLIAMS, J. F. AND MORRISON, W. R. *A Textbook of Physical Education*. W. B. Saunders Co., Philadelphia, 1939.

WILLIAMS, J. F., DAMBACH, J., AND SCHWENDENER, N. *Methods in Physical Education*. W. B. Saunders Co., Philadelphia, 1933.

WOOD, T. D. AND CASSIDY, R. *The New Physical Education*. The Macmillan Co., New York, 1931.